Examination Notes in Psychiatry

Basic Sciences:
A Postgraduate Text

Gin S. Malhi BSc(Hons) MBChB MRCPsych
*Social Genetic and Developmental Research Centre, Institute of Psychiatry,
and Maudsley Hospital, University of London*

Alex J. Mitchell BMedSci(Hons) MBBS MRCPsych
Department of Psychiatry, University of Leeds, and St James's Hospital, Leeds

ARNOLD

A member of the Hodder Headline Group
LONDON • NEW YORK • NEW DELHI

D0412356

This edition first published in Great Britain in 1999 by Butterworth Heinemann.

This impression published in 2004 by
Arnold, a member of the Hodder Headline Group,
338 Euston Road, London NW1 3BH

http://www.arnoldpublishers.com

Distributed in the USA by
Oxford University Press, Inc.,
198 Madison Avenue, New York, NY10016
Oxford is a registered trademark of Oxford University Press

Whilst the advice and information in this book are believed to be true and
accurate at the date of going to press, neither the authors nor the publisher
can accept any legal responsibility or liability for any errors or omissions
that may be made. In particular (but without limiting the generality of the
preceding disclaimer) every effort has been made to check drug dosages;
however, it is still possible that errors have been missed. Furthermore,
dosage schedules are constantly being revised and new side-effects
recognized. For these reasons the reader is strongly urged to consult the
drug companies' printed instructions before administering any of the drugs
recommended in this book.

British Library Cataloguing in Publication Data
A catalogue record for this book is available from the British Library

Library of Congress Cataloging-in-Publication Data
A catalog record for this book is available from the Library of Congress

ISBN 0 7506 4088 X

3 4 5 6 7 8 9 10

Printed and bound in India by Replika Press Pvt. Ltd.

What do you think about this book? Or any other Arnold title?
Please send your comments to feedback.arnold@hodder.co.uk

Contents

Preface

Candidates sitting the MRCPsych examination have consistently identified the basic sciences component as their Achilles' heel. There are several probable reasons why this is so.

Firstly, many of the basic science topics are difficult to define in terms of the extent of knowledge necessary for examination success. Secondly, for clinicians, the basic science topics perhaps appear to be less relevant to clinical practice and make less stimulating reading than the more familiar clinical topics. Consequently, they are perceived as being 'harder to learn'. Lastly, there are few books, if any, that provide comprehensive coverage of the basic science topics as relevant to the MRCPsych examination in a readable and memorable manner.

This book has been written with these points in mind and includes the essential basic sciences information needed for the MRCPsych examination. The format is such that further reading can be appropriately structured around this core information, however, so as to minimize the need to refer to other texts every attempt has been made to ensure that topics are covered in sufficient detail and are easy to understand. To aid memory there is ample use of mnemonics, diagrams and useful tables and appendices.

It is hoped that this book will be a useful tool for all those 'studying psychiatry' whether they are clinicans, those sitting examinations or indeed students.

Examination Guidance

The MRCPsych examination structure is under constant revision and it is best to obtain the most recent guidelines from the college at the time of application.

Probably the most common reason for failure is a lack of sufficient preparation and therefore it is important to begin preparing for the examination in good time. Many candidates prefer private study as this allows them to work at their own pace. Some draw motivation from working alongside others, for instance in study-groups. In addition most candidates attend some form of structured teaching and some may even attend specific examination courses. Unfortunately, in response to a common question; 'there is no "best way" of passing the examination'. All those sitting these examinations are essentially 'examination experts' having sat many important exams in their career. In most cases it is probably not advisable to make any dramatic changes to your individual style of preparation. However, the following suggestions may be of help.

1 Obtain the necessary *up to date texts* (see later) bearing in mind their relevance and readability. These are texts that you will have to read repeatedly and so it is important that you find them reasonably engaging.
2 Set aside *regular reading* and *revision periods*. These need not be onerous and it is amazing how much can be achieved simply reading 45 minutes per day, however, the key word is regular and ideally this much time should be set aside *every day*. This can then gradually be increased as the time of the examination approaches.
3 From the outset it is important to familiarize yourself with the standard of knowledge being tested by the examination. Attempt to gauge the level of understanding required by talking to those who have recently sat the examination and studying past papers.
4 Practice, under examination conditions, a complete paper or a portion of a paper when beginning revision. This will give you an indication of the areas that need further attention. It is less fruitful to do this near the time of the examination as there will be little time to correct your mistakes and learn new information. However, note that regular exposure to examination conditions and questions is essential throughout the revision period as this will fine tune your examination technique and reinforce learnt material.
5 It is important to manage your anxiety effectively. A modicum of anxiety is necessary in order to maintain motivation and assist in learning. However, overwhelming anxiety is counterproductive and can be prevented perhaps by having in place an achievable revision timetable and observing the above suggestions.

Finally, the MRCPsych examination is a difficult professional examination and, despite the inevitable bold claims of successful candidates, it is hard to imagine how anyone can pass the examination without making a deliberate effort. However, it is important not to panic and equally not to be lulled into a false sense of security. Instead, revise in good time, use whatever means necessary suited to your personal style of learning and above all be guided by your own experience and advice from experienced others.

Gin S. Malhi

Acknowledgements ·

We would like to thank Professor Iain Campbell, Professor Malcolm Lader, Professor Peter McGuffin and Professor Michael Reveley for their invaluable assistance and expert guidance.

1 *Basic psychology*

Learning theory

Learning is an experience based, relatively permanent change of behaviour, that is not the result of maturation or because of reversible influences such as drugs, hunger or fatigue.

Learning can take place through association, from observation or by understanding. Associative learning includes classical and operant conditioning.

Observational learning, also known as vicarious or social learning, involves modelling.

Cognitive learning involves understanding and concerns the use of cognitive strategies to process information.

Associative learning

Classical conditioning (CC) (respondent learning) Described by Pavlov (1849–1936) in 1927.

CC involves repeated pairing of a new stimulus with an **unconditioned stimulus** (UCS).

The UCS is known to elicit a specific **unconditioned response** (UCR).

The repeated association results in the new stimulus being able to produce the same response.

The new stimulus is the **conditioned stimulus** (CS) and the learned response is termed the **conditioned response** (CR).

Pavlov used food (UCS) to make dogs salivate (UCR) in response to a light or bell (CS).

The association is an **automatic behaviour** and does not require understanding.

The period of association between UCS and the CS is called the **acquisition stage** of conditioning. Acquisition of a CS is selective (easier to condition some stimuli than others) and the fact that some stimuli are more likely to become a CS than others is termed **stimulus preparedness**.

Learning a new CS through association with the original CS (which is now the UCS) is **higher order conditioning**. In **simultaneous conditioning** the CS and UCS are applied simultaneously (CS continues until response occurs) but this is less effective than **delayed conditioning** in which the CS precedes the UCS (optimal delay is 0.5 s). Least effective is **trace conditioning** in which before the UCS begins the CS has ended.

If the CS is repeatedly presented without the UCS then the CR gradually disappears, though not completely. This is called **extinction**.

If there is then a period of rest, during which the CS is not presented, the CR returns though it may be weaker than before. This is described as a **partial** or **spontaneous recovery**. The CR can also be recovered by repeating the association with the UCS.

The CR once established can be transferred to a stimulus that is similar to the CS even though the new stimulus has never been paired with the UCS. This is termed **generalization** and enables learning of similarities. Stimulus generalization diminishes in proportion to the novelty of the new stimulus.

Discrimination is the ability to recognize and respond to the differences between similar stimuli and it can be produced by differential reinforcement.

Repeated brief exposure to the CS results in an increase in the strength of the CR, this effect is termed **incubation**.

Using CC, **Watson** and **Rayner** in 1920 induced a white rat phobia in **Little Albert** (11 months old) by associating a noise with presentation of the rat. This was repeated with a white rabbit and generalized to any furry object.

Operant conditioning (OC) (instrumental learning) Skinner (1904–1990) proposed an associative learning theory based on **Thorndike's** (1874–1949) **law of effect**, which states that voluntary behaviour, involving **trial-and-error**, when successful is rewarded and strengthened and will therefore be repeated.

Skinner described two types of behaviour, respondent and operant.

Respondent behaviour is the consequence of known stimuli (e.g. neurological reflexes), whereas **operant behaviour** is independent of the stimulus.

In operant conditioning a hungry rat placed within a Skinner box (contains a lever which when pressed is associated with the release of food pellets) learns to press a lever (CR) which is rewarded by food. In this way the response is reinforced.

Primary reinforcement impinges directly on basic drives (e.g. nourishment, sex) and is independent of prior learning.

Secondary reinforcement (conditioned) derives from association with primary reinforcers and is based on prior learning (e.g. money, praise).

Reinforcement can be **positive**, in which a reward reinforces a response and increases the likelihood of its future occurrence, or **negative**, in which an unpleasant condition is removed and again increases the likelihood of the response. Negative reinforcement differs from punishment. **Punishment** is an aversive consequence that suppresses a response, reducing the likelihood of a future response. Punishment is most effective when it is prompt and able to suppress a response immediately. The removal of a punitive measure may allow it to act as a negative reinforcer. Punishment is one of three kinds of **aversive conditioning**. The remaining two are **avoidance conditioning**, in which the response prevents an aversive event occurring and **escape conditioning**, in which the learnt response provides complete escape from the aversive event which remains unchanged (this is extremely resistant to extinction). Aversive conditioning when performed in the imagination is termed **covert sensitization**.

In operant conditioning different **reinforcement schedules** lead to varying behavioural patterns. This is known as programming. Reinforcement intervals may be fixed or variable.

With **continuous reinforcement** (contingency reinforcement) the behaviour is quickly acquired and the response rate is at its maximum.

In **partial reinforcement** only a fraction of the responses are reinforced and this is more effective in maintaining behaviour and it is more resisitant to extinction; types of schedule:

- **fixed interval** reinforcement (poor at maintaining CR and the response rate increases at expected time of reinforcement);
- **fixed ratio** reinforcement (follows fixed number of responses) is effective in maintaining rapid response rate as reinforcement follows certain number of responses;
- **variable interval** reinforcement is effective in maintaining CR and response rate does not change between reinforcements;
- **variable ratio** reinforcement produces relatively constant rate of response since at any given time the likelihood of reinforcement remains relatively unchanged.

Shaping (successive approximation), based upon operant conditioning, involves reinforcing approximations to the desired behaviour so that in stages the latter is achieved. It is used in the management of those with learning difficulties where the desired behaviour is often infrequent or may be altogether absent.

Chaining is another technique occasionally used in people with learning difficulties. A desired complex behaviour is broken down into a series of simpler steps which are taught separately and then eventually linked together.

Premack's principle states that a high frequency behaviour can be used to reinforce a low frequency behaviour by making engagement in the former contingent upon satisfying some aspect of the latter.

Wolpe described **reciprocal inhibition** as a process in which an anxiety inhibiting response diminishes the connection between a stimulus and an anxiety response when it occurs in the presence of the anxiety-inducing stimulus. In the context of phobias it is maintained that opposing emotions cannot simultaneously coexist.

This then forms the basis of **systematic desensitization,** which involves gradual exposure in imagination or reality to the anxiety-inducing stimulus along a previously decided **hierarchy** from least to most. Immediate exposure to elements at the top of a hierarchy without any gradation of anxiety-inducing stimuli is called **flooding** when carried out *in vivo* and **implosion therapy** when accomplished through imagination.

Habituation is a form of adaptation which involves learning to respond selectively to novel stimuli as opposed to those that are constant and without serious consequences. **Sensitization** involves the strengthening of a response to a stimulus because of its significance.

Cognitive learning

Active learning involving the creation of cognitive maps which allow the formation of mental images and the development of structure and meaning.

Cognitive learning takes place either as **insight learning** (spontaneous cognitive remodelling that provides sudden insight or solution to problem) or **latent learning** (learning occurs but is not immediately apparent).

Observational learning: (vicarious or imitation learning, modelling)

Takes place through observation and may lead to the development of both classical and operant conditioning, though there is no direct reinforcement.

Effective models for observational learning:

- share features with observer (similarity)
- have high status
- are competent
- possess social influence/power.

Perception

Perception is an active process, the culmination of sensory and organizational functions, that produces meaning of the world.

Perception involves learning and as such is a developmental process.

Visual and auditory perception have been studied most.

Consciousness is buffered from crude information. Senses are specific and therefore the majority of information is not detected. That which is detected undergoes sensory processing prior to further modification centrally.

Gestalt principles of perception

From the Gestalt school of thought:

- Law of
  - **continuity:** interrupted line seen as continuous
  - **closure:** incomplete outline seen as whole
  - **proximity:** items juxtaposed grouped together
  - **similarity:** grouping of like items
  - **simplicity:** most basic precept is formed the sensory information available.
- Perception of the whole differs from that of the sum of its constituent parts. These parts are not divisible.
- **Figure ground differentiation**: the perception of figures from uniform background on basis of distinctive features.

Object constancy

The ability to maintain perceptual consistency in changing circumstances.

Several kinds of object constancy:

- colour/lightness constancy: object colour and lightness remain constant irrespective of lighting
- size constancy: object size remains constant irrespective of distance

- shape constancy: object shape remains constant irrespective of perspective (angle)
- location constancy: object position remains constant irrespective of viewer's motion.

Perceptual set

Responsive predisposition observed as a tendency to perceive and react to specific stimuli on the basis of expectation; hence

- reduction in the threshold of expected stimuli
- ambiguous stimuli perceived according to expectations and may undergo distortion/modification.

Influential factors; personality, experience, personal values.

Depth perception

To create 3D perception from a 2D retinal image the brain relies on several cues:

- monocular accommodation
- binocular vision and convergence
- object interposition
- object texture gradient
- linear and aerial perspectives
- relative size and brightness
- elevation and motion parallax.

Development of vision

Development of visual perception is based on interaction with the environment (constitutional–environmental interaction):

- birth: can discriminate levels of brightness*
              able to fix objects*
              able to track and scan objects*
              figure ground discrimination*
              poor visual acuity
              fixed focus (0.2 m)
- 1 month: differentiate faces (preference is shown for complex stimuli)
- 2 months: possess depth perception
- 4 months: colour vision and accommodation
- 6 months: accurate acuity (6:6).

(*Perceptual constancy, depth perception and object completion are acquired abilities as opposed to those that are innate and present at birth.)

Information processing

The derivation of meaning from sensory data. Processing can be data-driven or conceptually driven. Processing is mostly unconscious progressing in stages of organization and interpretation.

Data-driven processing

Prompted by data arrival and utilizing templates for pattern recognition and subsequent classification.

Conceptually driven processing

Insufficient data requires conceptualization of probable percept. Evidence is then sought in support of this possibility.

Attention

The selection of relevant information for further processing. Types of attention are:

Focused (selective) attention

One kind of information is selected for attention. **Dichotic listening** experiments show that alternative information *is* simultaneously processed and can be attended to if required.

Divided attention

Simultaneous attention is given to more than one source of information. Inefficient performance because of **dual-task interference**.

Controlled attention

Requires effort.

Automatic attention

Proficiency reduces necessary conscious effort.

Sustained attention

Performance progressively deteriorates.

Stroop effect

Interference of controlled process because of deeply rooted automatic processing.

Memory

Specific memories may be highly localized; however, memory function is largely poorly localized.

Memory is intrinsically linked to learning and involves:

- the learning of associations
- the learning of skills
- the storage of information
- the learning of new information (anterograde memory)
- the recall of previously learnt information (retrograde memory).

Memory process

- registration of information
- storage of information
- retrieval of information.

Registration/encoding

The initial processing of information enabling it to be assimilated (requires attention).

Storage

Multi-store model (Atkinson and Shiffrin) Sensory, short-term and long-term memory.

Sensory memory Large capacity but memories are unprocessed and of very short duration (<0.5 s). According to sense organ: echoic-auditory, iconic-visual and haptic-touch. It allows information to be processed, stored and assigned significance.

Short-term memory (STM) (primary/working memory) Temporary memory that allows conscious processing of information. Memory fades in 20–30 s unless rehearsed, typically, by repetition. Coding is primarily acoustic (visual encoding is very brief).

Finite capacity (7+2 units of information) that can be increased by chunking, i.e. the expansion of one unit to cover several by cognitively or perceptually introducing meaning, principle or formula and drawing similarities. Visual and verbal STM are stored in the R and L hemispheres respectively. Recall is error-free and effortless.

Long-term memory (secondary memory) Permanent store. Unlimited capacity (theoretically) limited by retrieval. Following registration needs few minutes for **consolidation**, i.e. without interference. Regardless of presentation information is stored and organized systematically and subsequent loss through forgetting is slow. Coding in LTM can be visual, acoustic and semantic and requires motivation. Storage and retrieval require effort (more than STM).

LTM can be declarative ('knowing that') or procedural ('knowing how').

Declarative memory can be episodic (knowing when) or semantic (knowing about).

Declarative-episodic LTM for events and places. **Autobiographical memory** that is clear and explicit.

Declarative-semantic (knowledge) Explicit LTM of meanings of words.

Procedural (non-declarative) *IMP*licit LTM concerning skills (*I*ntuition, *M*otor, *P*erception).

Retrieval

The recall of information from memory (LTM → STM).

Emotion influences LTM retrieval:

- facilitated by positive emotion because of increased rehearsal and organization
- converse with negative emotions/anxiety
- facilitated by reproducing original emotional context (**state-dependent learning**).

Primacy and recency effects Accurate recollection of an item is more likely if it is one of the first or last items to be learnt. **Primacy** because initial items receive most consolidation and **recency** because immediate information still in STM.

Explicit retrieval Memories are recalled completely with subjective temporal awareness.

Implicit retrieval No conscious recollection or temporal awareness. Behaviour indicates recall.

Forgetting

The loss of information from memory. Most often because of retrieval failure.

Two hypotheses for forgetting:

1 **Interference theory:** the learning and recall of an item is influenced by new learning in between as this disrupts consolidation of the original item (**retroactive inhibition**). Prior learning interferes with subsequent learning (**proactive inhibition**). Forgetting is item-dependent.
2 **Decay theory:** with time memories fade (trace-strength diminishes). Forgetting is time-dependent.

Levels of processing Structural; phonetic; semantic (Craik and Lockhart).

Motivation

Need–drive model

Needs produce drives which in turn motivate behaviour aimed at resolving
needs (goal-seeking behaviour). Needs – physiological, can be defined
objectively. Drives – psychological, hypothetical constructs.

Cannon's homeostatic drive theory

Change in homeostatic system triggers processes aimed at restoration of
system. Basic needs (biological needs), being self-regulating, function
homeostatically. To meet these intrinsic needs requires extrinsic
elements.

Extrinsic motivation theories

Hull's drive-reduction theory

Primary drives (basic, biological, innate drives) Necessary for
survival. Arise from homeostatic imbalance and result in arousal that
motivates behaviour (e.g. hypothalamic ventromedial nucleus – satiety
centre, ablation produces hyperphagia; lateral hypothalamus – hunger
centre, ablation produces aphagia).

Secondary (acquired) drives (Mowrer) Develop in association with
secondary goals through stimulus generalization and conditioning. Since
these are learned they vary considerably between individuals (e.g.
anxiety is a secondary drive).

Intrinsic motivation theories

Reduction of drive is not from external elements. Intrinsically motivated
behaviour is in itself gratifying or rewarding.

Optimal arousal Individuals strive for optimal level of arousal according
to their preference in order to achieve optimal performance. In general,
high and low levels of arousal lead to sub-optimal performance
(**Yerkes–Dodson curve**).

Cognitive consistency Festinger's theory: incompatible cognitions
held simultaneously or beliefs that are inconsistent with behaviour
cause dissonance which the individual is then motivated to resolve by

altering one of the parameters (cognition, belief, behaviour). The desire for cognitive consistency can therefore be considered a need (see Chapter 2).

Need for achievement (McClelland)

Need for achievement (cognitive model of motivation) relates to 'need' for self-ideal. Failure to match ideal results in drive to achieve. Eventual mastery results in pleasure. Personal **competence**, intrinsically rewarding, and involves desire for stimulation (as opposed to reduction as in homeostatic mechanisms) which can be achieved through: *COMPEtence*

Curiosity
Others (need to cooperate, reciprocate)
Manipulation
Play
Exploration

Maslow's (1908–1970) hierarchy of needs Combines extrinsic and intrinsic elements.

Hierarchy of needs (pyramidal form) ordered according to survival value. Those that are lower in the hierarchy must be satisfied before subsequent (higher) needs can be addressed.

Needs

Self-actualization   realize potential

Aesthetic   symmetry, beauty, order

Cognitive   understanding, exploration, knowledge

Esteem   social approval, competence, recognition

Belonging and Love (social)   affiliation, membership

Safety   safety, security

Physiological/Physical   thirst, hunger

Emotion

Emotions

Classified as eight primary emotions by Plutchik; from which juxtaposed emotions give rise to secondary emotions. Primary emotions seem to be universal whereas secondary emotions are culturally diverse.

Primary emotions	Secondary emotions
disgust anger	$\Rightarrow$ contempt
anticipation joy	$\Rightarrow$ love
acceptance fear	$\Rightarrow$ submission
surprise sadness	$\Rightarrow$ disappointment

Components of emotional response

– subjective awareness (cognition)
– physiological response
– behaviour.

Interaction of these results in emotional response.

James–Lange theory (1922)

Perception of an emotion-arousing stimulus causes physiological changes (visceral and skeletal) which along with behaviour are mentally interpreted and experienced as the relevant emotion. The emotion is therefore secondary to physiological responses.

However, criticized because:
– emotional changes faster than physiological response
– pharmacological induction of physiological responses not accompanied by appropriate emotion
– same physiological response can accompany opposing emotions.

Cannon–Bard (thalamic) theory

Perception of emotion-arousing stimulus leads to the concurrent experience of emotion and physiological responses. Thalamus controls processing of stimulus information and following its perception stimulates the cortex to produce appropriate conscious emotion and via the hypothalamus produces relevant physiological changes (visceral and skeletal).

Schacter's cognitive labelling theory

The conscious experience of emotion depends upon the stimulus, the physiological responses and cognitive appraisal. Circumstances, situational cues and cognitive factors can influence conscious emotional experience and this has been shown in studies.

Stress

Stress occurs when perceived resources are exceeded or overwhelmed by perceived demand or expectations (stressor). The individual's appraisal is of key importance. Responses to stress are determined by situational factors and the individual's psychological and physiological attributes.

Situational factors

Life events, daily hassles, daily uplifts, severe difficulties, conflict, catastrophe and trauma. **Life events** – significant happenings that result in change. Ranked according to impact and degree of associated stress. Applicable world-wide across cultures, life events show relation to many illnesses.

Physiological aspects

Stress can cause or exacerbate many illnesses (e.g. heart disease and enteric ulceration). Physical illness may itself be a stressor.

Psychological aspects

Stress can cause anxiety and depression, PTSD and aggressive behaviour. Alternatively, optimal degree of stress can enhance performance.

Stress response

Hans Seyle described the non-specific physiologic response to stress as the general adaption syndrome:

– alarm
– resistance
– exhaustion.

Vulnerability and invulnerability

Reaction to stressors determines susceptibility to stress-related illnesses.

Type A Behaviour pattern (personality): **DISTRAC**tible

*D*riven
*I*mpatient
*S*trive for *S*uccess
*T*ime urgency
*R*arely *R*elax
*A*mbitious and *C*ompetitive

NB relationship of type A personality and coronary heart disease.

Type B Do not possess these characteristics.

Invulnerable individuals Perceive changes/stressful events as challenges and have greater sense of control over their lives.

Coping mechanisms

Conscious responses used to counter stress. Can be problem- or emotion-focused. Problem-focused responses attempt to modify stressor or its effect. Emotion-focused responses attempt to alter individual's reaction without changing stressor.

Locus of control

Dimensional concept concerning perceived control over life. **Rotter** identified two loci of control:

Internal locus Relates to feeling of control over one's life and being responsible for personal behaviour. This is associated with healthy response to stress.

External locus Relates to opposite, i.e. feeling that life is externally controlled and determined. This is associated with a poor response to stress.

Learned helplessness

Learned generalized expectation of helplessness illustrated first by Seligman using dogs. Forms part of cognitive model of depression.

2 *Social psychology*

Attitudes

Evaluated beliefs that can

1 define social groups
2 establish identities
3 influence thought and behaviour.

Attitudes have several specific functions: **SKIVE**

Social adjustment – facilitate sense of belonging to a community
Knowledge – facilitate understanding of the world
Instrumental – practical or pragmatic
Value-expressive – express values
Ego-defensive – preserve self-esteem and shield from anxiety

Attitudes predispose an individual to behave in a particular manner. They comprise three components (***A,B,C***) which in theory influence each other. However, because of situational variables measured attitudes are often unable to predict behaviour:

an **A**ffective component (most resisitant to change) – feelings towards attitude object
a **B**ehavioural component – actual response/interaction with attitude object
a **C**ognitive component – beliefs concerning attitude object

Measurement of attitudes

Direct methods of measurement:

1 **Thurstone scale:** consists of statements that have been ranked and assigned values. Subject selects those that they agree with and a mean score is derived. Disadvantages: bias in ranking; different sets of responses can nevertheless result in same score. (NB it is not in itself an attitude scale but a method by which to devise one.)
2 **Likert scale**: comprises a number of statements and for each the subject indicates degree of agreement/disagreement on a five-point scale. This is more sensitive than the Thurstone scale but still different patterns of responses can result in same score.
3 **Semantic differential scale:** this consists of nine or more paired bipolar adjectives and for each there is a seven-point visual analogue scale on which the subject marks their response. This scale is easy to

use and has good test–retest reliability. However, it is difficult to interpret midpoint responses and there may be a positional response bias.

Direct measures are susceptible to social desirability bias. Subject offers 'expected' answers as opposed to genuine responses. Can detect the likelihood of this happening by using a lie scale and tendency can be diminished by emphasizing anonymity or embedding questions within irrelevant items.

Indirect methods can be used to assess attitudes but interpretation is difficult: physiological responses (e.g. Galvanic skin response); projective tests.

Other important methods for assessing attitude:

1 **Borgadus social distance scale:** measure of racial prejudice. It involves the selection of statements from a range representing degrees of social distance.
2 **Sociometry:** subjects in groups nominate preferred partners and create sociograms which identify sub-groups.
3 **Interview:** open-ended or structured.

Attitudes

Attitudes tend to predict behaviour best when:

1 strong and consistent
2 based on subject's personal experience
3 related specifically to the predicted behaviour.

Attitude change

Cognitive consistency is the desired endpoint of processing cognitive elements and forms the basis of several theories of attitude change. The desire for cognitive consistency can also be considered a basic need and so forms part of motivation (see separately).

Cognitive consistency theories Attitudes are linked so that one idea affects the way we respond to another.

1 **Heider's balance theory:** individuals seek harmony of attitudes and beliefs and evaluate related things in similar manner.
2 **Festinger's cognitive dissonance theory:** when an individual's behaviour is inconsistent with their attitudes this produces dissonance,

which then causes a change of attitudes so that they are consistent with behaviour. Dissonance is a negative drive state, characterized by psychological tension or discomfort, causing increased arousal which the individual attempts to reduce by:
- altering behaviour
- dismissing dissonance creating information
- developing and adding new explanations or ideas in favour of thoughts that are consonant.

Attitude change is also a means of reducing dissonance.

The degree of dissonance is in proportion to the perceived importance of the cognitions involved.

Increased dissonance occurs when:
- there is little pressure to comply
- the perceived choice is high
- there is an awareness of personal responsibility for any consequences
- consequences of any alternative behaviour are anticipated to be unpleasant.

Predictions of theory are counter-intuitive, imprecise and only partly supported empirically.

3 **Osgood and Tannenbaum's congruity theory:** when two attitudes or beliefs are mutually inconsistent the one that is less firmly held will change.

Persuasive communication

Applies to many situations, e.g. doctor–patient interactions and advertising.

Persuasion is dependent upon characteristics of the source (communicator, doctor), the message and the audience (recipient, patient).

Persuasive communicators

Possess a *RANGE* of characteristics:

1 *R*ecognized opinion leader
2 *A*udience is able to identify with communicator through similarity and/or communicator is *A*ttractive/likeable
3 *N*on-verbal cues facilitating communication (e.g. optimal proximity to audience)
4 *G*enuine motivation and having no vested interest in message
5 *E*xpertise and credibility

Recipient factors

1 Intelligence: curvilinear relationship.
2 Self-esteem: when low the use of simple messages enhances compliance.

Complex messages are persuasive in intelligent recipients with high self-esteem.

Message

*I*mplicit message more persuasive for *I*ntelligent recipient, explicit message more apt for less intelligent recipient.

Interactive personal discussion is more persuasive than impersonal one-way mass media communication.

One-sided One-sided uncritical presentation better suited to less intelligent audience and those who already favour message.

Two-sided presentation better suited to better informed, intelligent audience, particularly if neutral towards message.

Fearful message better at influencing recipients with low levels of anxiety, and the converse applies to those with high levels of anxiety (low fear message is better).

Type of persuasion determines kind of **attitude change**:

- **Identification**   based on attraction to or admiration of communicator.
- **Internalization** based on belief in claims, i.e. message.
- **Compliance**   based on punishment/reward and not really a change of attitude.

Interpersonal attraction

Individuals seek others for friendship and companionship. Interpersonal attraction which is a facet of interpersonal perception is enhanced by several factors: ***PARCELS***

*P*roximity/*P*ropinquity; dependent upon degree of intimacy and culture bound interpersonal space
*A*ttractiveness (physical)
*R*eciprocal self-disclosure
*C*ompetence (perceived)

*E*xposure (familiarity)
*L*iking (reciprocal)
*S*imilarity: particularly significant in the beginning and early part of a
   relationship. It is more important than complementarity (becomes
   increasingly important with time) and remains so.

Theories of interpersonal attraction

Exchange theory Preference for relationships that offer greatest gains
(reward) with least expense (cost).

Equity theory Added factors of investment, and constancy, in gauging
rewards and costs of a relationship. The relationship should be 'fair'
with approximately equal gains in the long run.

Proxemics Interpersonal space (body buffer zone) is determined by
personal factors and cultural rules and mediated by non-verbal cues.
Different body parts vary in terms of availability for contact (gender and
relationship of those involved is also important): hands>arms/face>
trunk/legs>pelvic region.

Some individuals have larger personal space, e.g. schizophrenics and
violent criminals (particularly behind themselves). Initially respond
violently to intrusion of this and then withdraw.

Matching hypothesis (similarity hypothesis) Pairing of individuals
(to form romantic partners) results in them being closely matched in
terms of their mutual rewards. Usually, a partner of similar physical
attractiveness is sought.

Attribution theory

Attribution is the process of interpreting the behaviour of others. It is a
cognitive process concerned with behavioural causality.

Individuals tend to attribute their own behaviour to situational (external)
causes but that of others to dispositional (internal) causes. This bias in
attributing the behaviour of others is called the **fundamental (primary)
attribution error**.

Self

An individual's *self* or *self-concept*, as described by Carl Rogers, consists of all the perceptions, values, attitudes and ideas that they have concerning themselves. It does not necessarily reflect or correspond to reality. Separate from this is the *ideal self*, which is all that the individual would like to be.

Social influence

Social facilitation

Task performance is enhanced by the presence of others. Facilitation is not necessarily because of competition as others can simply be observers (**audience effect**).

However, with new or complicated tasks or hostility from others, performance may decline.

Bibb Latane proposed a **Social *I*mpact *T*heory** (***SIT***) stating that in any particular setting the degree of social influence is a function of the:

*S*trength
*I*mmediacy and
*T*otal number of people exerting the influence

In social situations of urgency **bystander intervention** is affected by **pluralistic ignorance** and **diffusion of responsibility**.

Social power

Influence over others exerted by individuals or groups. Five methods/types are described by French and Raven: ***RACER***

*R*eward: influence is derived from being able to reward
*A*uthority: (legitimate) influence is derived from status or role
*C*oercion: influence is derived from ability to punish (usually implied)
*E*xpertise: influence is gained by demonstrating skills or knowledge
*R*eferential: influence is because of charisma, being liked and admired

Conformity

Yielding to group pressure by way of persuasion or example such that there is a change in attitude or behaviour.

Informational social influence: individual conforms to group ideas and behaviour outwardly and privately.

Normative social influence: conforms outwardly but privately maintains own opinion.

Solomon **Asch** experiments. Used confederates (accomplices, stooges) in small groups to attempt to alter the opinion of an individual assessing line length. Naïve subject shown to be significantly influenced by confederates' incorrect answers.

To avoid social rejection the subject agrees with the group view even when their own personal opinion differs.

Conformity increases with:

- group number (maximum effect with **three** confederates)
- perceived high status of other group members.

NB conformity diminishes greatly if even a single member of the group agrees with subject.

Vulnerability to conform is less in those that are:

- self-reliant
- intelligent (high IQ)
- socially able
- expressive.

Obedience

Milgram (Stanley) conducted experiments involving the administration of potentially fatal shocks by subjects, under the instruction and supervision of an expert (experimenter), to protesting subjects (stooges) who were in fact part of the experiment and acting accordingly. He was able to show that the subject's obedience was **increased** by:

- perceived authority of experimenter
- presence of experimenter
- belief in 'contract' with experimenter
- distancing from distressed and protesting subject.

Subjects' obedience stems from:

- acceptance of experimenter's sense of right and wrong
- inability to challenge experimenter's morality because of ensuing social awkwardness.

Zimbardo (Philip), using college students in mock prison, similarly showed that unwillingness to express moral concerns could lead to tolerance of escalating brutality.

Leadership

Leadership characteristics dependent upon:

- task requirements
- group characteristics
- development (pathway of emergence)
- influence ascribed by role.

Distinction of three *Le*A*D*ership styles (by Lewin):

*L*aissez-faire
*A*utocratic
*D*emocratic

Table 2.1 Leadership styles

Style	Laissez-faire	Autocratic	Democratic
Interaction within group	Aggressive	Aggressive	Cooperative liking
Interaction with leader	Detached	Submissive and attention-seeking	Task-related
Absence of leader	Abandon task	Abandon task	Continue independently
Task completion	Poor	Good	Good
Effectiveness	Creative tasks	Urgent tasks	

Fiedler's contingency theory Fiedler (Fred) correlates leadership style (measured using LPC) and task/group characteristics.

Degree to which leaders distinguish between least and most preferred co-workers gives rise to scale and scores of least preferred co-worker (LPC).

High LPC score Person is **relationship-orientated** and perceives least preferred co-worker in relatively favourably. Considerate and accepting in relationships.

Low LPC score Person is **task-orientated** and strongly disapproves of least preferred co-worker. Dominant and controlling in relationships.

Proposes that high and low LPC leaders suited to different types of tasks and that this is influenced by relationship with group members (see Table 2.2).

Table 2.2 Contingency theory

Task	Relationship with group	Best leader
Structured	Good	Low LPC
Unstructured	Good	High LPC
Unstructured	Poor	Low LPC

Groups

Group decisions tend towards consensus, with individuals suppressing opposing opinions so as to avoid dissension. This is described as **groupthink**. It occurs in situations where there is:

– pressure to conclude
– prominent opinionated leader
– cohesive group shielded from outside influence.

It results in inadequate exploration of alternatives.

When individuals express their opinions separately and then group to decide upon the same matter, the eventual outcome is likely to be more extreme than that of the group average. This is termed **polarization** and occurs partly because of reinforcement.

In groups the individual behaviour of group members is less important than that of the whole group. This suppression of individuality is termed **deindividuation**.

Intergroup behaviour

Ingroup: any group with which a person identifies.

Outgroup: any group with which the person has an association but does not identify.

Stereotypes: generalizations concerning individuals or groups of people involving characterization using specific features on the basis of assumption and inference. However, stereotypes are usually constructed around some facts and as such are exaggerations or simplifications. Once established stereotypes are difficult to change and become self-fulfilling as fresh observations are biased by the working stereotype so that only supportive information is selected.

Prejudice: prejudged, unjust and biased attitude derived from incomplete knowledge. It is usually a negative attitude that is resistant to change.

Prejudice stems from:

- personality factors (authoritarian)
- differences in attitudes and beliefs
- the use of stereotypes.

To reduce prejudice there should be:

- an environment supporting equality
- the attainment of equality
- the opportunity for personal contact
- contact with non-stereotypes
- collaborative endeavour.

Group membership Leads to biases of social perception:

- outgroup is perceived as being homogenous*
- ingroup is perceived as being heterogenous*
- members of ingroup are perceived more positively.

(*NB reciprocal applies if ingroup is the minority group.)

Aggression

Behaviour to harm.

Instrumental aggression Aim is to gain reward or cause suffering.

Hostile aggression Aim is to injure.

Theories of aggression

Ethological theories Aggression is innate. Behaviour that diminishes aggression:

- distancing self
- familiarity with aggressor
- evoking conciliatory response.

Operant conditioning The consequences of aggression determine the likelihood of repetition. Gains (physical, psychological, social) act as positive reinforcers.

Psychoanalytical theories Consider aggression to be a basic instinct.

Social learning theory Aggression is learned through modelling. Experimentally shown observation and imitation of aggressive behaviour.

Frustration-aggression hypothesis Failure to achieve causes frustration. Frustration is intimately linked with aggression and aggressive drive precipitates aggressive behaviour. Aggression can be directed towards the source of frustration or displaced. However, although experimentally frustration most often leads to aggression it can instead cause emotional disturbance or apathy. Emotional arousal increases aggressive behaviour, possibly through classical conditioning.

Media Viewing television violence increases aggressive behaviour but only in boys (social reinforcement).

Correlates of aggressive behaviour Characteristics of parents and family associated to an individual's aggressive behaviour:

- Family: large
           lower socio-economic group
           lack of positive emotional expression.
- Parents: young; aggressive
           physical punitive measures
           inconsistent or permissive in parenting.

Interpersonal cooperation

Altruism Extreme form of helping behaviour in which the interests of others are given importance. Strictly applied there should not be any perceived personal gain. Generally, helping behaviour is not completely unselfish. Altruism is a form of defence mechanism permitting the resolution of conflicts.

Social exchange theory Behaviour is driven by the expectation of reward. Regarding helping behaviour the expectation is that of future reciprocity.

Interpersonal cooperation Cooperation usually applies in circumstances where:

- without cooperation a specific aim cannot be fulfilled
- another party also has the same aim
- the aim is not exclusive (i.e. can be fulfilled simultaneously by more than one party).

In such situations cooperative behaviour is influenced by:

- number of parties involved (with increasing number cooperation diminishes)
- prior knowledge of other parties
- behaviour of other parties
- extent of communication between parties
- possible pros and cons of various actions undertaken.

Neuropsychology

Language

Left hemisphere shows dominance: 99% of R-handed and 60% of L-handed individuals.

Areas of importance for language:

Broca's area (motor speech area); Broca, Paul (1824–1880)

Located in the inferior frontal gyrus (opercular/triangular zones) (BA 44 and 45). It coordinates the production of coherent speech.

Wernicke's area (receptive language area); Wernicke, Carl (1848–1905)

Consists of auditory association cortex located in superior temporal gyrus (BA 22 and 42). It makes sense of language.

Angular gyrus (BA 39)

Interconnections with association cortices.

Damage affects ability to read and write.

Neuronal circuits

speech → auditory/association cortices → Wernicke's area
  → **comprehension of speech**

speech ← motor regions ← Broca's area ← Wernicke's area
  ← mentation

text → visual/association cortices → angular gyrus → Wernicke's area
  → **reading and understanding**

writing ← motor regions ← angular gyrus ← Wernicke's area
  ← mentation

Speech and language defects (dysphasias)

Speech defects involve frontal, temporal and parietal lobe damage. Location and extent determine type of dysphasia:

Fluency Fluent dysphasia involves regions posterior to sylvian fissure. Converse for non-fluent.

Table 3.1 Dysphasias

Term	Explanation	Location in L hemisphere
Semantics	Meaning of words	Temporal lobe
Phonology	Language sound-pattern	Superior temporal
Syntax	Grammar	Anteriorly
Prosody	Intonation emotional content	Anteriorly right* hemisphere

(*exception)

Comprehension Damage to Wernicke's area results in difficulty with comprehension.

Naming Affected in all aphasias.

Repetition Affected by lesions to peri-sylvian region (includes Wernicke's and Broca's areas and arcuate fasciculus connecting them). Transcortical (motor/sensory) syndromes show sparing of repetition.

Expressive aphasia (Broca's) Damage disrupts higher control of muscular articulation (though they are functionally normal) such that fluidity of speech is diminished (slow, effortful) and words are mispronounced or approximated (phonemic paraphrasias). Agrammatism reduces speech to telegraphic style with paucity of functional words such as prepositions. These deficits (speech and syntax) are usually partial. Comprehension of speech and written language remain intact though the ability to write may be affected.

Receptive aphasia (Wernicke's) Damage results in fluent incoherent speech containing neologisms (content is abnormal). Speech is effortless

Table 3.2 Summary of aphasias

Aphasias	Comprehension	Naming	Repetition	Fluency
Fluent-				
Wernicke's	●	●	●	
Conduction		●	●	
Anomic		●		
Transcortical-sensory	●	●		
Non-fluent-				
Transcortical-motor		●		●
Broca's		●	●	●
Global	●	●	●	●

(● = impaired)

and without dysarthria. Grammatical structure is largely maintained though some unusual syntax is produced (paragrammatism). Naming is profoundly impaired and individuals are unable to repeat words and are often unaware of any communication difficulty. Writing and reading are also affected.

Conduction aphasia Damage to supramarginal gyrus containing arcuate fasciculus, the main connection between Broca's and Wernicke's areas. (Often occurs during recovery from Wernicke's.) Comprehension and verbal fluency unaffected; however repetition is severely impaired.

Transcortical aphasia Can be motor or sensory and arise because of cortical/sub-cortical damage outside of peri-sylvian language regions. Repetition is preserved.

Anomic aphasia Caused by localized dominant angular gyrus damage.

Anomia is marked and distinctive in this syndrome, which is usually manifest during recovery from other aphasias. NB Anomia is a poor localizing sign.

Global aphasia Combines features of other aphasias occurring because of total left hemisphere dysfunction.

Thalamic aphasia Dominant thalamus lesion. Presentation similar to sensory transcortical aphasia.

Basal ganglia aphasia Hemiparesis is accompanied by comprehensive difficulties and dysarthria.

Aprosody The non-dominant hemisphere is responsible for the insertion and interpretation of the emotional inflexions of speech. Non-dominant frontal lobe lesions affect this function as language is received and produced.

Other cortical cognitive functions

Agnosia

Inability to understand or interpret the significance of sensory information in spite of intact sensory pathways and sensorium. Agnosias indicative of sensory association area lesions.

Types of agnosia

Visual agnosia Inability to recognize by visual inspection alone a previously identifiable object. Cf. anomia – individual unable to name object but *can* describe its use. Individual with visual agnosia can do neither.

Caused typically by lesions in BA 18 and 19 occipital lobe. L-sided lesions – agnosia for colours and objects. R-sided lesions – agnosia for spatial relations.

Agrapghagnosia (agraphaesthesia) Unable to identify figures (numbers/letters) drawn on palm, aka tactile agnosia.

Autotopagnosia Inability to recognize, name or identify (by pointing) own body parts upon request. Cf somatagnosia – inability to identify own or other's body parts.

Finger agnosia Inability to recognize individual fingers, seen in Gerstmann's syndrome.

Astereognosia Inability to recognize (form, shape) objects by palpation.

Simultanagnosia Able to grasp individual aspects but not overall meaning of a picture.

Colour agnosia Can perceive colours but unable to correctly name them.

Hemisomatognosia Individual feels that a limb that actually exists is absent.

Prosopagnosia Unable to recognize faces. (NB mirror sign in Alzheimer's disease).

Anosodiaphoria Lack of concern about neurological deficit.

Anosognosia Failure to recognize or appreciate deficits or disease. Lack awareness, especially of hemiplegia.

Apraxia

The inability to perform volitional acts in spite of intact motor system and sensorium.

Types of apraxia

Constructional apraxia Inability to draw shapes, construct figures or geometrical patterns.

Ideational apraxia Unable to perform coordinated sequence of complex movements.

Dressing apraxia Unable to dress.

Oral (orobuccal) apraxia Unable to perform skilled, learned facial, tongue and palate movements.

Ideomotor apraxia Unable to perform progressively harder tasks.

Alexia Loss of the ability to read. Cf. dyslexia; developmental reading difficulty.

Agraphia Loss of the ability to write.

Frontal lobe

Frontal cortex of humans is uniquely enlarged and the most recently developed part. The frontal lobes make up a third of cerebral hemispheric mass and the prefrontal cortex forms 30% of total cortex of brain. Specific areas:

- motor area; takes up pre-central gyrus
- pre-motor area; anterior to motor area (BA 6 and 8)
- dorsolateral area; (BA 9, 10, 45, 46)
- basomedial area; (BA 9-13, 24, 32).

Dorsolateral and basomedial areas are often grouped together as prefrontal region.

Frontal eye field is a specialized area located in posterior portion of middle frontal gyrus (BA 8).

Cortical granular layers II and IV determine granularity/agranularity of cortex. Motor cortex agranular (BA 4, 6) also parts of BAs 8 and 44. Remaining cortex anterior to this is granular.

Connections of prefrontal cortex (PFCx) with dorsomedial nucleus of thalamus (dmN.Th)

Magnocellular region (medial part of dmN.Th) → → basomedial area (orbital and medial regions)

[damage can cause pseudopsychopathic syndrome]

Parvicellular region (lateral part of mdN.th) → → dorsolateral area

[damage can cause psuedodepressive syndrome]

Neurological disorders involving frontal lobes

- neoplasms (90% of brain tumour patients presenting with psychiatric symptoms have frontal lobe involvement)
- cerebrovascular diseases
- multiple sclerosis
- trauma
- degenerative diseases.

Motor and pre-motor cortex

- Function:
  - motor control (primary and secondary levels)
  - fluency (verbal and design)
  - spelling.
- Lesion effects:
  - motor: contralateral spastic paresis; loss of fine motor control
  - fluency: reduced (particularly verbal)
  - spelling: impaired.
- Others: *GROUPS*

  *G*egenhalten (opposition)
  *R*eflexes (primitive) – grasp reflex; glabellar tap; pouting; palmo-mental reflex; suck reflex; snout
  *O*ptic atrophy (ipsilateral)
  *U*rinary incontinence
  *P*erseveration
  *S*eizures (Jacksonian)

Prefrontal cortex

Intellectual functions: *SPACE*

*S*equencing (ordering tasks)
*P*rocessing (mental agility)
*A*ttention
*C*oncentration
*E*xecution

Any of these can be impaired in frontal lobe damage.

Personality changes:

pseudopsychopathic *CDEFGH*

*C*hildish excitement (**moria**)
*D*isinhibition
*E*uphoria
*F*amiliarity
*G*arrulousness
*H*umorous punning (**Witzelsucht**)

pseudodepressive *RAPID*

*R*etardation (psychomotor)
*A*pathy
*P*lacidity
*I*ndifference (lack of concern)
*D*rive *D*iminished (lack initiative)

4 *Psychological assessment*

Principles

A good test should be:

- reliable
- valid
- discriminatory
- standardized.

It should preferably be:

- easy to administer
- cost-effective.

Scaling

This involves the transformation of data in accordance with a scale. The scale is based on some ascertainable/measurable characteristic (parameter) of the data and in this respect there are several types of scale (structural differences):

Nominal

Qualitative data, categories for classification, not suited to statistical analysis and individual scores have no alternative value or meaning. Group can be described by mode, frequency or proportion.

Ordinal

Scores along scale are placed in rank order at varying intervals and have relative but not absolute value and only signify order giving no indication of difference. Group can be described by range and median.

Interval

Ordinal scale with scores separated equally. No absolute zero but uniform intervals allow derivation of both order and difference. Group can be described by arithmetic mean and variance.

Ratio

Akin to interval scale with uniform intervals but in addition possess absolute zero and therefore possess absolute value. Group can be described by geometric mean and coefficient of variation.

Scales can also be distinguished according to purpose.

- Discriminatory (differential) scales: provide groups or categories. Can be used for classification or diagnosis.
- Descriptive (intensity) scales: measure extent or severity.
- Prognostic scales: measure course and outcome.
- Selection scales: predict outcome following specific treatment.

Methods of assessment

Ratings using scales Can be conducted by:

- respondent (self-report)
- interviewer (observation or interview).

Errors of assessment

- central tendency: bias towards centre avoiding extremes
- leniency error: tendency to select extremes
- response set: tendency to always agree or disagree with questions
- logical error: rating items that have some 'logical link' in similar fashion (treating them as a group)
- Hawthorne effect: presence of interviewer alters the situation and influences responses
- Halo effect: answers are selected so as to fit with other responses
- social acceptability: respondent gives expected answers (those believed to be expected by interviewer). Can be reduced by use of forced-choice or false items.

Norm-reference

A standard score for a group/population is termed the norm. This is then used for comparison. This approach allows the results from different studies to be compared to the population norm and to each other.

Criterion-reference

This serves a similar purpose to norm-referencing. However, the standard, termed the criterion, is selected more arbitrarily often chosen such that comparison allows assessment of performance on a particular test. Criteria should be unbiased, reliable and relevant.

Validity

The extent to which a test or scale measures 'what' it intends to measure is described as validity. It is a relative term and can be expressed as a correlation between that which is measured and the desired attribute. There are several types of validity:

Content validity Extent to which all aspects of the subject matter are assessed.

Face validity Whether the intended characteristic appears to be measured (subjective appraisal).

Criterion validity Measures ability of test or scale to distinguish subjects already known to differ on the basis of an external, validated measure. It is of two types:

Concurrent validity Comparison of simultaneous measures involving reference to an external valid measure.

Predictive validity Ability to predict outcome as measured now and in the future or on another scale.

Cross validity The extent to which the criterion validity of a measure is retained when applied to a new set of subjects.

Incremental validity Extent to which a new measure approximates to true validity offering additional benefit and improving on other measures.

Construct validity Relates to the purpose of the measure and relies on establishing both convergent and divergent validity:

Convergent validity This assesses the degree of association between measures that are expected to be closely correlated. Correlation is assumed because they measure the same property.

Divergent validity The degree to which a measure discriminates that being assessed from unrelated measures.

Reliability

The reliability of a test/measure indicates the degree to which it can be replicated and describes the extent of agreement amongst repeated assessments. There are several types of reliability:

Inter-rater reliability The degree of agreement between different raters assessing the same parameters within the same time-frame.

Intra-rater reliability The degree of agreement between assessments made at different times by the same raters assessing the same parameters.

Split-half reliability Signifies the internal consistency of a test/measure. It describes the extent to which equivalent components (two halves) of the test/measure correlate when compared.

Test–retest reliability Signifies the stability of a test/measure. It describes the degree of correlation between two assessments conducted under identical conditions but at different times.

Sensitivity

The degree to which a test/measure is able to detect/identify the property that it determines (positive results).

Specificity

The degree to which a test/measure is able to distinguish and exclude those without the property that it determines (negative results).

Predictive value (PV)

Positive PV The proportion correctly described by a test as positive (i.e. possess sought parameter).

Negative PV The proportion correctly described by a test as negative (i.e. lack sought parameter). See also Chapter 16.

Intelligence

Various definitions based on different parameters can be used to define and describe intelligence (no one definition is universally accepted).

- Galton – attempted to measure intellect (created instead the correlation coefficient).
- Spearman – developed concept of general intelligence factor (g).
- Thurstone – proposed primary mental abilities: **MNOPQRS**

   Memory, **N**umber, w**O**rd fluency, **P**erceptual speed, verbal **Q**omprehension, **R**easoning, **S**pace

- Hebb – type A (genetically based potential), type B (effective intelligence).
- Cattell – fluid ability and crystallized ability.
- Sternberg – component intelligence (deductive ability and verbal reasoning: used for executive tasks) and experiential intelligence (automation of routine tasks permitting attention to be focused on new learning).

Intelligence is best characterized according to that being assessed: **ABCD**

Assessment approach

- **psychometric methods**: define specific and general abilities examining for instance visual and verbal factors of intelligence. Performance correlates between specific factors, however, it is difficult to define the number of necessary specific factors.
- **computational methods**: examine the information-processing involved in problem-solving. Five components are suggested (Sternberg): **TRAMP**

   Transfer; **R**etention and **A**cquisition components, which deal with transfer of knowledge, memory and learning; **M**eta-components, which decide upon selection of strategies; and **P**erformance components, which carry these out

Biological aspects

Cultural aspects

Developmental aspects

Definition of terms

General factor of intelligence (g) Thought to be substrate of general intelligence underlying intellectual functioning.

Fluid intelligence That which is used for novel situations/problems. Basis of initiative and creativity.

Crystallized intelligence Relies on prior learning and use of previous experience/knowledge.

Attainment Achievement, consequence of learning.

Aptitude Potential ability.

Mental age (MA) Measure of intellectual ability devised by Binet.

Intelligence quotient (IQ) Percentage ratio involving mental (MA) and chronological age (CA):

$$IQ = \frac{MA}{CA} \times 100$$

Assessments are designed so that average MA score equals CA providing a mean IQ of 100 (standard deviation 15). Intelligence is assumed to have a normal distribution.

Measured intelligence increases up to 16 years of age. Plateau from 16 to 25 years of age with subsequent gradual decline until 5 years prior to death, when there is a significant decline in IQ (terminal drop).

Intelligence tests

Adults

Wechsler Adult Intelligence Scale (WAIS) For those aged 16 years and over.

Consists of 6 verbal and 5 performance subtests providing verbal and performance IQs

Verbal: *SAD VIC*

*S*imilarities
*A*rithmetic
*D*igit span
*V*ocabulary
*I*nformation
*C*omprehension

PerfOrmance: *ABCD*

*O*bject assemby
picture *A*rrangement
*B*lock design
picture *C*ompletion
*D*igit symbol

The addition of all the scores provides a full scale IQ.

National Adult Reading Test (NART) List of words with unusual pronunciation. Represents pre-morbid IQ.

Mill Hill Vocabulary Test Based on recognition and recall.

Raven's Progressive Matrices Involve diagram completion. Different tests for different age groups. Do not rely on recall of information and are easy to use. Missing pattern piece of a matrix is selected and from the raw score a percentile is derived. Therefore less sensitive to cultural differences and can be used for those with communication difficulties.

Children

Stanford–Binet Intelligence Scale From age 2 years. Tests short-term memory and reasoning (verbal, quantitative, abstract, visual). IQ is derived by comparison with normative data.

Wechsler Pre-school and Primary School Intelligence Scale (WPPSI) From ages 4 to 6½ years. Verbal and non-verbal.

Wechsler Intelligence Scale for Children (WISC) NB Revised (WISC-R)

From 5 to 15 years. Verbal and non-verbal.

Intelligence tests are affected by:

- individual factors: culture, anxiety, motivation
- situational factors: interaction with assessor (e.g. hostility)
- test factors: age specificity (children especially), function/purpose specificity

Contentious findings concerning intelligence

- Inappropriate use has led to erroneous interpretations, e.g. IQ variance according to racial differences.
- Intelligence has an inverse relationship with:
  - increasing family size
  - birth order.
- Positively associated are:
  - inheritance (of intelligence)*
  - education.
  (*Heritability of intelligence is a controversial issue; however, the closer the biological relationship the closer the IQs approximate.)
- Studies show that the IQ of children is related to:
  - home life-style
  - education
  - perseverance.

NB not particularly related to parental wishes or social class.

Boys have greater range of intelligence than girls.

Personality development and assessment

Theories of personality development

Nomothetic (nomological) Based on population studies and concerned with the structure of personality (trait and type theories).

Ideographic (radiological) Based on study of the individual and concerned with aspects of individuality (personal construct, humanistic and psychoanalytic theories).

Kelly's personal construct theory Man's interpretation of the world is scientific. Based on personal experience each individual formulates various **constructs** that allow them to make predictions. Each individual's 'system' of constructs, both conscious and unconscious, organized in an hierarchy provides a sense of identity. Having to negotiate outside the scope of personal constructs gives rise to anxiety.

Roger's self theory Every person strives for fulfilment and tries to cultivate an **ideal self**. Most important is congruence between the person's perception of themselves and reality and their self-image in comparison to the ideal self. Anxiety stems from behaviour not in keeping with one's own self-image. Individuals able to attain and maintain such congruence are able to self-actualize, achieve and be successful in both psychological and social aspects of their personality.

Bannister's repertory grid Uses bipolar constructs to asses attitudes.

Erikson's theory of psychosocial development Requires the successful resolution of a crisis at each stage of development. Erikson emphasizes concepts of identity (inner preserving sense of sameness), identity crisis and identity confusion. Epigenesis refers to the stages of ego and social development.

(Cf Freud's psychosexual stages of development.)

Table 4.1 Psychosocial development

Age	Crisis	Successful outcome
0–18 months	Trust/mistrust	Sense of security/attachment
18–36 months	Autonomy/doubt	Self-control/efficacy
3–6 years	Initiative/guilt	Confidence
6–12 years	Competence/inferiority	Competence
12–adulthood (adolescence)	Identity/confusion	Achieve self-identity
Adulthood	Intimacy/isolation	Commitment
Middle-age	Generativity/stagnation	Concern about others
Maturity	Integrity/despair	Fulfilment

Erik Erikson (born 1902, Montessori teacher) adopted Freud's structural and topographical models and agreed that development is biological, i.e. genetically determined. Disagreed with psychosexual emphasis. Freud emphasis on Id; *E*rikson emphasis on *E*go.

Categorical versus dimensional approaches to personality

Categorical approach places people in separate categories (e.g. Kretsch-mer's and Sheldon's associations with body-build). Dimensional approach characterizes personality in terms of degrees (extent or intensity) of traits (e.g. Eysenck's and Cattel's theories).

Kretschmer Linked personality and body-build as follows:

- athletic (muscular): outgoing, robust
- asthenic/leptosomatic (lean): solitary, self-conscious, cold, aloof, self-sufficient, schizothymic
- pyknic (rounded and stocky): relaxed, sociable, cyclothymic, variable in mood

Sheldon Made similar types of links:

- mesomorphy (muscle, bone): somatotonia, show energy and assertiveness
- ectomorphy (fragility): cerebrotonia, prefer symbolic expression
- endomorphy (soft roundness): viscerotonia, prefer enjoyment, relaxation

Eysenck's personality theory Derived the following dimensions from factor analysis of rating scale data: neuroticism–stability; extroversion–introversion; psychoticism–stability; intelligence.

Cattel's trait theory Derived 16 first order personality factors (PF) and Cattel's 16PF test from factor analysis of thousands of words describing personality. Subsequent second order analysis of these provides three dimensions: intelligence, anxiety, sociability. (NB similar to Eysenck's dimensions.)

Measurement: Maudsley Personality Inventory (MPI); Eysenck Personality Inventory (EPI) and Eysenck Personality Questionnaire (EPQ). Latter is most recent development. It assesses psychoticism and contains a lie-scale.

Psychometric assessment of personality

Objective tests e.g. EPQ; Minnesota multiphasic personality inventory (MMPI) – commonly used self-report inventory.

Respondent has limited options. Mental state significantly interferes with scoring hence semi-structured interviews and observer-based ratings preferred.

Projective tests Based upon the presentation of an ambiguous stimulus to which the individual responds in keeping with personality, e.g. Thematic Apperception Test (TAT); Rorschach Inkblot Test.

5 Human development

Stage theories

Development occurs as a series of progressive stages. Each is necessary for the occurrence of subsequent maturation. The sequence of stages is constant and environmental influences can only alter the rate of development. Transitions between stages are described as **critical periods**.

Progression through stages and critical periods is driven by **maturational tasks**. These tasks allow the development of more complex behaviours. The culmination of developmental processes is termed **maturity,** which can therefore be described more specifically as physical, intellectual or sexual maturity.

Attachment

Attachment theory

Infants increasingly focus on one or more individuals. This natural behaviour is genetically determined and is necessary for subsequent development. When one individual is chosen this is termed **monotropic** attachment.

Attachment is infant to mother (*c*hild → *m*other). Bonding is mother to infant.

Attachment behaviour Is that displayed by the infant towards the **attachment figure** (the focus of such behaviour), usually but not necessarily the mother. Attachment behaviour depends on affection. In an attachment figure contact, comfort and warmth are sought even in preference to food (**Harlow**'s wire mother monkey experiments).

Age (mth)	Attachment behaviour
<6	infant seeks care through closeness but is indiscriminate in attachment
6	monotropic attachment accomplished
12	emergence of fear of strangers
36	attachment figure can be substituted

Lorenz explained attachment as form of **imprinting**. Imprinting occurs in animals other than primates.

Secure attachment behaviour Prominent during first three years of life (6–36 months).

- Attachment figure (AF) separation causes distress and anxiety.
- Upon return of AF infant seeks contact/comfort from AF.
- Infant uses AF as secure base from which to explore environment intermittently returning to base to seek reassurance and comfort.

Secure attachment depends upon:

- temperament of infant
- AF nurturing
- AF encouraging independent exploration
- AF providing secure base.

Secure attachment lays foundation for initiative and formation of relationships.

Insecure attachment behaviour

	Avoidant	Ambivalent
In absence of AF	muted clinginess	excessive anxiety
Upon return of AF	little or no reaction	reluctance to engage

Insecure attachments may lead to difficulties in establishing relationships, and disorders of childhood and adolescence. Avoidant attachment may lead to aggressive behaviour later in life.

Separation

Separation before 6 months or after 3 years age has little effect. This then is the critical period during which separation leads to (after Bowlby):

- protest: crying and searching for AF
- despair: as AF has not returned
- detachment: indifference to AF.

Prolonged separation (maternal deprivation) is associated with: ***ABCDE***

*A*ttention-seeking and *A*ggressive behaviour
*B*onds are difficult to make and sustain (easily *B*roken)
*C*old, un*C*oncerned behaviour
*D*evelopmental language delay and *D*warfed growth
*E*nuresis

Family relationships

Parenting

Involves various components described as:

- nurturance (P → C)
- communication (P ↔ C)
- control(P → C) and
- maturity demands (P → C).

Parenting style can be categorized as:

- authoritative: nurturing parents with high expectations and strict rules
- authoritarian-restrictive: less nurturing but still quite controlling
- permissive: unconditionally nurturing.

Different styles of parenting result in different characteristics of children.

Distorted family function (dysfunctional families)

Exhibit: *CORE*

*C*ommunication problems
*O*verprotection: of members of family, aspect of enmeshment; excessively close
*R*ejection: weak attachments within family and parents under-involved; loneliness
*E*nmeshment: over-involved parents stifle child's individuality

Exclusive relationships within the family (triangulation) can also cause discord as can scapegoating children for marital discord.

Intrafamilial abuse

Most damaging in early childhood as this is time of greatest vulnerability and developing personality. Abuse can be physical, sexual or both.

Sequelae common to both forms of abuse:

- **d**epression and anxiety states
- **d**issociation
- **d**isordered personality – borderline personality disorder
- **d**istrusting and paranoid traits
- **d**ependence on defence mechanisms (denial, splitting).

Physical abuse (NAI-non-accidental injury)

Sequelae:

- Are themselves aggressive, may suffer impairments (neurological, cognitive) and delays in development.
- Are likely to repeat abusive behaviour towards own children.

Sexual abuse

Sequelae: *SHAME*

*S*exual impulses more difficult to control and sexual identity is weakened
*H*omosexuality is more likely
*A*lcohol and drug abuse
*M*olestation of children is more likely
*E*ating disorders

Abuse (physical and sexual) in the long term causes diminished self-esteem and a predisposition to self-harm.

Divorce

Parental divorce is almost invariably associated with some degree of distress to children. Usually this is self-limiting (up to a year) and the outcome is dependent upon the:

- child's temperament and age at time of divorce
- nature of the divorce (amicable, hostile)
- relationships between siblings and between children and parents
- degree of communication
- parents' abilities to adjust and make provisions for the children.

Temperament

Temperament refers to the basic dimensions of personality thought to have a biological basis and appear early in life.

One study (Thomas and Chess) described nine aspects of temperament which were then grouped together as follows when studying the interactions of children and their parents:

(A third could not be easily categorized.)

- **Easy child (40%)**
  - regular in habits (eating, sleeping)
  - adaptable to change/novel situations

- emotional stability
- positive and responsive to new stimuli.
- **Difficult child (10%)**
  - irregular in habits
  - slow or unable to adapt
  - emotional lability
  - negative and unresponsive to novel stimuli.
- **Slow-to-warm-up (40%)**
  - slow to adapt
  - suspicious of novel situations
  - poor response to new stimuli, often withdraw.

Cognitive development

Piaget's model

Jean Piaget (1896–1980), having observed his own children, proposed that a child's cognitive development is dependent upon interaction with its environment and that this progresses at varying rates through specific stages. Children think differently (qualitatively) to adults and are often unable to distinguish or separate their personal perspective (**egocentrism**). Intelligence involves understanding and inventing new ways of interacting with the environment.

schema	refers to cognitive structure or pattern of behaviour/ knowledge
assimilation	refers to the incorporation of new or novel information into existing thought patterns (schemas)
accommodation	refers to the adjustment or modification of existing schemas so as to facilitate comprehension of new information (which has not been achieved by use of existing schemas alone)

Therefore:

New experience outside of existing schemata ⟶ Disequilibrium which prompts

Equilibrium   *circular reaction*

Assimilation ⟵ New schemas ⟵ **Accommodation**

Piaget described four stages:

(NB ages for the following stages are only approximate)

Sensorimotor stage (0–2 years) Child has innate reflexes that are modified by functional exercise. Develops causal relationships between self and outside world. However, does not understand temporal relationships and thoughts exhibit egocentrism.

4 months – primary decentring; detaches self from external environment. Develops discriminatory smiling.

8 months – purposeful behaviour commences.

12 months – begins to develop object permanence (hidden object still exists).

Pre-operational stage (2–7 years) Precausal logic; animism; symbolic stage.

Child uses deferred imitation (symbolic play, drawing) and acquires components of language. Thought involves: ***AMPLE*** ('ample thought')

*A*nimism: characteristics of life are attributed to all objects
authoritarian *M*orality: rules are sacrosanct, bad-doing should inevitably be punished
*P*recausal *L*ogic: non-scientific, based on child's internal world
*E*gocentrism

Occasionally divided into **pre-conceptual** (2–4 years) and **intuitive** (4–7 years).

Concrete operational stage (7–11 years) Myelination of the CNS is complete at age 7 years. Children lose animism, authoritarianism and egocentrism. A second decentring of thoughts occurs enabling development of logical thought. Are able to perform **operations** such as those involved in comprehending the **laws of conservation**.

Aspects of thought that take prominence are as follows: ***LOGIC***

*L*ogic
*O*perations (mental manipulation of thoughts)
*G*roup activity/cooperation
*I*dentity and *I*ndividuation of thought (but understand other person's point of view)
*C*omprehend *C*onservation (reversibility)

Formal operational stage (11 years and upwards) Beginning of hypotheticodeductive thought, involving the complex manipulation of ideas and the application of sophisticated reasoning: ***ABCD***

*A*bstract (propositional) thought
*B*elief systems

Conceptualization
Deductive reasoning

NB this stage may not necessarily be attained even by adulthood.

Language development

- Language – the requisite skills for communication
- Phoneme – essential unit of sound
- Morpheme – meaningful units of sound (words). Contain phonemes
- Semantics – meaning
- Syntax – grammar

The acquisition of language and the learning of communication skills can be affected by a variety of factors.

Table 5.1   Stages of language development

Age	Language development
3 months	Babbling (series of phonemes)
9 months	Repetitive babbling; imitate mother's speech acts
12 months	Speaks three words
18 months	Speaks any one of 18–40 words
24 months	Vocabulary >240 words. Grammatically pairs words. Telegraphic speech
36 months	Early comprehension of grammar and syntax
48 months	Correct use of grammar. Language comprehension better than expression
60 months	Language akin to adult speech

Language is slower to develop:

- **biological**
  - in boys
  - with intrauterine growth retardation
  - following a prolonged second stage of labour
  - in twins
  - because of a lack of stimulation (deaf).
- **environmental**
  - in large families
  - in those from social classes IV and V
  - because of a lack of stimulation (neglected).

Kohlberg's theory of moral development

Kohlberg proposed six stages of moral development grouped as three
levels on the basis of having presented stories posing moral dilemmas to
a variety of subjects.

Level I: preconventional morality

- stage 1: punishment
- stage 2: reward

Level II: conventional morality

- stage 3: approval/disapproval
- stage 4: authority

Level III: post-conventional morality

- stage 5: social contract
- stage 6: personal principles/ethics

Though there is some correlation between age and moral level, many adults
may not reach level III. Levels I and II can be loosely correlated to Piaget's
preoperational (2–7 years) and concrete operational (7–11 years) stages
respectively. Level III is usually broached in adolescence.

Social perspective-taking

This is the ability to adopt 'another person's point of view', being objective
and able to detach opinion. It is a precursor of empathy and moral
reasoning. Prerequisites are adequate cognitive and moral development
and a robust sense of personal identity.

Childhood development of fears

Fear is by definition an unpleasant experience that is prompted by a
perceived danger (imminent or ongoing). Infants are generally fearless
and most fears are acquired/learnt.

Fears can be learned and maintained by both classical and operant
conditioning. Some fears are more easily acquired (**stimulus preparedness**), perhaps because of an evolutionary genetic predisposition. Fears
can also be developed and sustained by social learning and modelling.

Table 5.2 Development of fears

Age	Fears	
Newborn	Visual cliff	
6–12 months	Darkness; height	
12 months–3 yr	Strangers; separation	Increasing
3–6 yr	Learn fear responses; animals	severity of
6–12 yr	Social shame	stimulus
Teenage onwards	Failure; illness; death	
Adulthood	PTSD	↓

Sexual development

Embryology

Gonads initially appear as gonadal ridges (week 5). Primordial germ cells appear in gonadal ridges 1 week later (week 6). Gonads acquire morphological characteristics week 7. A significant reduction in the number of primordial germ cells is thought to have a masculinizing effect. This can be because of an over-ripe ovum at the time of fertilization as this is associated with a decrease in the number of primordial germ cells.

Sex is determined by the chromosomes carried by the germ cells. XY → male; XX → female.

Y chromosome carries testis-determining factor (SRY gene) and results in indifferent gonads developing medullary cords (testis) and tunica albuginea and suppressing the development of the cortical cords (ovary).

The gonads release hormones which influence further sex differentiation and the development of external genitalia.

Testis stimulate mesonephric ducts to form vas deferens and epididymis. Testicular androgens stimulate formation of penis, scrotum and prostate.

Ovaries stimulate paramesonephric ducts to form uterus, uterine tubes and upper one-third of vagina. Oestrogen stimulates the formation of labia, clitoris and lower two-thirds of vagina.

Definitions

Sexual identity Refers to biological status as male/female.

Gender identity Person's self-awareness/perception as male/female. Usually gender and sexual identity correspond but in case of transsexual the two do not agree.

Gender role Masculine and feminine behaviours corresponding to gender that identify individual as male/female (stems from gender role stereotypes).

Sex/gender typing Differential treatment of different sex children. Influences acquisition of gender identity and gender role.

Sexual orientation/preference Preference regarding sexual partner. Heterosexual (opposite sex partner), homosexual (same sex partner) and bisexual (either/both).

Sexual drive Basic need for sexual gratification.

Gender identity development Usually achieved by age 5 years. Possible developmental theories:

- Cognitive: less than age 5 years understanding of gender is incomplete. Cognitive development increases self-awareness and after age 5 years children have usually developed perception of their gender and associated role.
- Psychoanalytical: Freud's theory of sexual development. Through repression and identification children acquire gender role having negotiated Oedipal/Electra complexes.
- Social learning: children acquire self and gender identity by modelling and then internalizing learnt social and gender behaviours.

Sexual orientation Debate concerns whether innate (biological determinism) or learnt. Tentative findings concerning sexual orientation/preference:

- established prior to puberty (fairly early) and sexual activity
- parental interaction/influence and nature of initial sexual experience are of little determining importance.

Adolescence

Puberty

Changes associated with the development of reproductive ability.

Described as primary (concern sex organs) and secondary sexual changes:

- Males: average onset 11.5 years of age. Initially there is an increase in size of the testis and then the penis and the appearance of pubic hair. There is also a change of body proportions, an overall increase in size, the appearance of facial hair and the lowering of vocal pitch.
- Females: average onset 11 years of age. Commences in most cases with breast development but in some (20%) begins with pubic hair growth. First menses (menarche) occurs on average age 13–14 years.

Conflict

Conflict with authority is a feature often associated with puberty/ adolescence. Culturally this view is more representative of Western societies.

Possible explanations for conflict during this period of growth:

- ethology: conflict forces adolescent to adapt and forge role, identity, purpose
- separation–individuation: expectancy (societal) and desire (personal) for ongoing dependence (on authority/parents) conflict with ability to be socially independent
- cognitive development: intellectual maturation prompts alternative initiatives which may differ from or oppose traditional views
- Erikson's psychosocial development: adolescent seeks to create personal identity and achieve autonomy.

NB many adolescents undergo its transitions without significant conflict.

Affective stability

There is a slight increase in emotional instability during adolescence. This is due to both psychosocial and biological changes that accompany this period. Adolescent affective instability tends to remain in adulthood.

Adaptations in adult life

Adaptation continues throughout life. Common adaptations include: pairing and parenting.

Pairing

The development of a permanent romantic relationship has a positive effect on mental and physical health (i.e. stable fulfilling relationship is protective and promotes health).

The selection of a suitable partner is influenced by several factors:

- attitudes: partners tend to come from similar cultural background and have similar socio-economic status
- partners that offer best cost–benefit ratio are preferred (social exchange theory) [preferred relationships are those in which both partners feel equity in this process are (equity theory)]
- attractiveness: seek similar level of attractiveness even though would desire a more attractive person than oneself (matching hypothesis). Imbues sense of security as individual feels less likely to be rejected.

Different cultures place differential emphasis on certain attributes. Men from most cultures rate physical attractiveness highly while women place greater emphasis on drive and economic success.

Parenting

Parenthood affects both the parents and their relationship.

Fathers and mothers adopt more 'feminine behaviours'.

The relationship between parents usually becomes more affectionate despite possible stresses (reduced income, sleep, personal space and time).

Good parenting (affectionate, caring and supportive) enhances the child's self-esteem. Bad parenting (abuse, neglect) increases the likelihood of later problems.

Illness

Acute illness is a common stressor, prompting concern about socio-economic future. Likelihood of illness and coping strategies change with age. Chronic illness leads to adjustment in stages:

- shock: sense of disbelief
- encounter: react by grieving and possibly becoming depressed
- retreat: use denial to avoid dealing with illness or its consequences
- intrusion: gradual adaptation and acceptance of fate.

Grief, bereavement and loss

Grief

The affective, behavioural and cognitive concomitants of bereavement. Typical grief involves (cf. illness):

- initial sense of disbelief and shock
- emotional arousal as loss becomes apparent
- denial of anger
- biological symptoms of depression, e.g. sleep disturbance, changes of appetite and weight
- identification with deceased.

Bereavement

The process following the loss of a loved person through death.

Stages of bereavement:

Protest initially in a state of shock: stunned and feeling numbed
Preoccupation involves yearning with subject of loss – illusions and hallucinations; some symptoms of depression
Disorganization manifest denial and sometimes irritability
Resolution eventually come to terms with loss; accept and adjust to reality.

NB bereaved more likely to consult their family doctor and at increased risk of dying during first 6 months.

Indicators of poor resolution or adjustment:

- loss of child, spouse
- loss is sudden, 'out of the blue' or traumatic
- occurs at time of additional stresses
- from poorer socio-economic background
- ambivalent/dependent relationship with deceased.

Typically grief resolves within 6–12 months.

Mourning

The voluntary social expression of loss.

Ageing

Ageing brings about physiological and psychosocial changes.

Physiological

Physiological functions decline at varying rates: notably – vision, hearing, new learning, decision-making. However, some cognitive functions may improve (e.g. memory) because of practice or experience.

Psychosocial

Psychosocial changes are even less predictable. Stigma attached to ageing (particularly in Western societies). More likely to be lonely. Social isolation (sensory decline/deficits; less likely to socialize; fewer friends). Sexual drive and enjoyment may remain intact but socially not accepted. Individuals become less neurotic and more able to contain emotionality.

Death and dying

The realization of imminent or impending death may lead to the following phases (after Kübler-Ross):
  – denial: disbelief; refusal to accept reality; reject diagnosis
  – anger: 'why me'; attach blame-bargaining; attempt to negotiate better outcome
  – bargaining: attempt to negotiate in return for a cure
  – depression: outpouring of feelings; may become clinically depressed
  – acceptance: resolution of above phases; calm and understanding.

Adjustment to death involves both the dying individual and family and friends. Good communication and affection help both the patient and those around them to adapt.

⑥ Social sciences

Definitions

Social class

A population sub-group defined by relatively stable social parameters:

*M*oney (financial wealth)
*O*ccupation/income
type of *R*esidence and its location
*E*ducational achievement

Essentially the *MORE* you have the higher your **socio-economic status**. NB unlike some other social systems (e.g. the Hindu caste system), there is potential mobility between classes through educational and financial means.

The Registrar-General's classification, introduced in 1911, divides society into six social classes that form a hierarchy. In Britain social class is primarily based on occupation and decided according to the head of a household. The social classes are labelled O, V, IV, III, II and I: unemployed, unskilled, semi-skilled, skilled, intermediate and professional, respectively.

Psychiatric disorder and social class

Socio-economic status is a very strong predictor of morbidity and the relationship extends to psychiatric disorders. The reasons for this may be:

- social causation theory: the greater environmental stress and increased adversity experienced by those belonging to lower social classes contributes in some way to the development of psychiatric ill-health.
- social selection/drift theory: those with psychiatric illness are not equipped to remain in the higher social classes and so either remain in the lower social classes or gravitate towards them.
- differential treatment/labelling: race and social class bias the management of those with psychiatric illnesses producing a misrepresentation.

Psychiatric illnesses more commonly diagnosed in the lower social classes are:

- alcohol dependence
- schizophrenia
- depression
- illicit drug abuse
- psychopathic.

Those more commonly diagnosed in the higher social classes are:

- bipolar affective disorder
- eating disorders.

Social class and psychiatric healthcare

The utilization of psychiatric healthcare services has been described by Goldberg and Huxley as a series of five levels, each of which equates to a stage along the route of assessment and care. Movement from one level to the next entails passing through a filter, and there are four such filters which have to be negotiated successfully in order to gain access to the final level. The levels and filters are:

- **Level I:** The community
  Filter 1: Illness behaviour prompting decision to seek help
- **Level II:** GP attenders
  Filter 2: Detection of disorder by GP
- **Level III:** Diagnosed as ill
  Filter 3: Decision as to whether specialist help is needed
- **Level IV:** Specialist service attendees
  Filter 4: Decision to hospitalize
- **Level V:** Specialist service in-patient

Decisions as to when and how individuals move through a healthcare system are based on:

- characteristics of the service: funding, waiting lists, geographical convenience etc.
- nature of the disorder: severity, risk to patient and others etc.
- social aspects of the individual: age, gender, race, status etc.

Psychiatric patients from poorer socio-economic backgrounds are more likely to:

- become psychiatric in-patients
- remain as in-patients for longer periods of time
- be subjected to physical treatments such as ECT.

These health inequalities were highlighted by the 1980 **Black Report** which examined health in relation to social class. It reported that, in relation to those from social class I, individuals from social class V:

- have double the neonatal mortality
- are twice as likely to die prior to retirement
- have an increased rate of most diseases.

Reasons proposed for these inequalities are:

- good health promotes an improvement in social class; poor health a decline
- economic power determines ability to 'purchase' good health; e.g. materials-food, residence and lifestyle
- disease promoting behaviours more strongly associated with the lower social classes, e.g. smoking.

The doctor–patient relationship

Doctor's role

An individual's pattern of social behaviour is their **social role.** For doctors and patients Parsons put forward a model incorporating their obligations and rights.

A doctor's social role is:

- to diagnose and define illness
- to offer support and treatment
- to legitimize illness and patient sick role.

Doctors therefore confer the **sick role** which gives the patient certain rights and places them under certain obligations:

- rights: exempt from blame, i.e. not responsible for having illness
                 excused from usual/normal duties, e.g. household activities or work
- obligations: to desire recovery and to seek necessary help
                 to cooperate in the assessment and management of their illness.

Illness behaviour

Mechanic defined illness behaviour as 'the ways in which given symptoms may be differentially perceived, evaluated and acted upon'.

Abnormal illness behaviour has been defined by **Pilowsky** as 'the persistence of a maladaptive mode of experiencing, perceiving, evaluating and responding to one's own health status'. The illness behaviour is disproportionate to the underlying disease (real or not).

There is tendency for doctors caring for those with abnormal illness behaviour to focus on somatic symptoms, often leading to inappropriate treatment which may inadvertently reinforce the abnormal behaviour.

Psychiatric disorders and families

There are important interactions between some of the major mental illnesses and aspects of family life.

Schizophrenia

Theories originally thought to contribute to the aetiology of schizophrenia:

- Disordered communication; double-bind and abnormal family communication.
- Abnormal (deviant) role relationships; schizophrenogenic mother and martial schism/skew.

Double-bind (Bateson) Abnormal parental communication during childhood generated ambivalence. Messages conflicting, incompatible and vague causing confusion and ambiguity. Child receives 'contradictory injunctions' from which there is no satisfactory escape. Originally thought to precipitate withdrawal, irrational behaviour and eventually schizophrenia.

Abnormal communication (Wynne and Singer) Suggested that abnormal family communication (non-sequential, disrupted) led to schizophrenia in offspring.

Schizophrenogenic mother (Fromm–Reichman) Specific maternal characteristics lead to schizophrenia in offspring: *HORtID*

*H*ostile
*O*verprotective
*R*ejecting
*I*ndifferent
*D*istant

Marital schism/skew[Lidz]

- Schism – parental division because of conflict splits child's loyalties.
- Skew – dominant, intrusive mother and submissive, compliant father leads to maternal eccentricities dominating family life and these intrude into child's life causing disturbance.

Expressed emotion Expressed emotion (EE >35 hours per week) better predictor of risk of relapse than compliance with medication. EE is characterized by; critical comments, hostility and emotional over-involvement. Reducing exposure to EE, medication and appropriate family intervention can reduce the effects of EE. Hence importance of educating family about illness, engaging patient in activities outside of family sphere, e.g. work or attendance at day hospital.

Alcohol abuse and dependence

Drinking excessively leads to a variety of problems (violence, psychological distress/disorders, the abuse of other substances, financial loss). These have a detrimental effect on family relationships.

Depression

Vulnerability factors relating to women, identified by early research (Brown and Harris): maternal loss before 11 years of age, having three or more children below the age of 15 years, lack of employment outside the home and the lack of a confidante.

Life events

Major life events (LEs) have serious negative implications and produce lasting change (technically a LE can be positive or negative but in psychiatric context latter is usually implied).

LEs can be assessed by Holmes and Rahe Social Readjustment Rating Scale (self-report questionnaire) or Life Events and Difficulties Schedule (LEDS). Latter is a more reliable and valid measure which entails a semi-structured interview.

Relationship between LEs and psychiatric disorders

Schizophrenia LEs significant in terms of relapse and course of illness but not instigation/onset.

Depression Severe abuse (violent, sexual, emotional) during childhood is related to development of depression. LEs four times more likely to have occurred (as compared to those without depression) in year prior to depressive illness. Losses (material and psychological) are of particular importance, leading to feelings of low self-esteem, humiliation, hopelessness and entrapment. Suicide attempts are even more often preceded by significant LE.

Puerperal psychosis Studies show little relationship with LEs, particularly in patients with previous psychotic illness.

Mania Association with LEs unclear.

Institutions

Generally contain a selected population. They have rules and routines and so can lead to problems of understimulation, isolation, loss of independence, skills and status. These changes because of institutionalization can lead to diminished motivation, apathy and social withdrawal.

Social institutions are those in which members have agreed forms of relationship (e.g. families). **Total institutions**, however, have very many individuals, isolated from the outside world for a considerable length of time, living together in a regulated manner (e.g. prisons, traditional psychiatric hospitals).

Goffman highlighted the disadvantages of institutions such as large psychiatric hospitals and described institutionalization and institutional life.

Important terms that Goffman used:

- **binary living and binary management**: staff appear to live in a different world to that of the patients they manage;
- **batch living**: in institutions the normal components of life (working, home life and leisure) are often absent;
- **mortification process:** the process of becoming an inhabitant of a total institution. It begins with the **betrayal funnel** (relatives send the patient to hospital with the help of health professionals) and involves **role-stripping** (admission to hospital – removal of personal effects, 'stripping' for physical examination, bathing and being given 'new' clothes) and adoption of **patient role**.

Goffman also described the reaction of patients to the process of mortification:

- rebellion, withdrawal, pretence to compliance (colonization), conversion, institutionalization.

Many of those who showed withdrawal had additional symptoms (submissiveness, apathy, diminished self-esteem and an inability to plan) that Barton grouped under the syndrome of **institutional neurosis**.

'The three mental hospitals study' (Netherne, Mapperley, Severals) found that the extent of clinical poverty (poverty of speech, social withdrawal, blunted affect) in schizophrenic patients was associated with the poverty of their social environment.

Prejudice

The adoption of an attitude on the basis of insufficient information such that a preconceived set of beliefs are formulated and maintained. Though technically prejudice can be negative or positive, in practice it is the negative meaning that is usually applied. Prejudice often involves the use of group stereotypes and may arise because of differences of attitude and belief. Discrimination, the application of prejudice, can be on the basis of any attribute, for example sex (sexism), race (racism) or age (ageism).

Explanations for prejudice:

- Cultural approach:
  realistic conflict theory – the struggle of more than one group competing for common resources results in cohesion of the groups and inter-group hostility.
- Motivational approach:
  authoritarian personality
  frustration-aggression theory – frustration from one source is displaced and expressed as aggression.
- Cognitive approach:
  stereotyping-development of defective beliefs about other groups.

7 *Important theorists and their concepts*

Sigmund FREUD (1856–1939)

Influenced by:

- Helmholz (distribution of energy and modelling psychological theories upon physical ones)
- Brucke (concepts of conservation and energy)
- Meynert (linked neuroanatomy to behavioural consequence)
- Charcot (initial work on hysteria and hypnosis strongly affected Freud)
- Hughlings Jackson (from whom theories relating to association and regression are derived).

Freud developed several theories:

- theory of hysteria (published *Studies on hysteria* (1895) in conjunction with Breuer)
- topographical theory of the mind
- structural theory of the mind
- theory of dreams
- theory of psychosexual development.

Topographical model

Earliest model, described in *The interpretation of dreams* (1900), and consists of three parts:

1 Conscious Awareness of external and internal perceptions:

- involves secondary process thinking
- governed by the reality principle
- content is readily available/accessible.

2 Preconscious Acts as a censor (between unconscious and conscious) withholding that which is unacceptable.

Develops during childhood (parallel to the development of the ego).

Like conscious, involves secondary process thinking and is governed by reality principle.

Content can be brought into consciousness through selective attention.

3 *Unconscious* All mental processes outside of consciousness. Repressed ideas, memories, feelings and urges:

- entails **primary process** thinking
- governed by the **pleasure principle**
- information is only accessible provided preconscious is 'disabled' or compromised, e.g. during dreaming censor is relaxed.

Table 7.1   Primary and secondary process thinking

	Primary process thinking	*Secondary process thinking*
Time	Timelessness	Linear forward flow of time
Organization	Lacking	Systematized
Reality	Disregard of conscious world reality	Regard for external reality
Logical connections	Disregarded	Regarded and respected
Contradictions	Are not recognized	Acknowledged but not always accepted
Tolerance for inconsistency	High	Low
Governing principle	Pleasure	Reality

The **pleasure principle** is largely innate and involves the seeking of pleasure and the avoidance of pain:

- it is the immediate gratification of instinctual drives leading to wish fulfilment.

The **reality principle** involves delayed gratification and is the result of external reality.

Structural model

Described in 'The ego and the id', this model supplanted the topographical model. Freud divided the mind into three components:

1 *Id* Unconscious reserve of impulses, drives, instincts. These basic drives concerning aggression, survival, sex etc. dominate thinking (primary process) according to the pleasure principle. It is non-verbal, illogical and has the following components:

- eros: life instinct, creative force
- thanatos: death instinct, destructive and aggressive elements
- libido: derived from the id, manifests initially as ego libido (primary narcissism) and then object libido.

2 Ego The ego is the integrator; it is that part of the personality that mediates with the external world. A large proportion is conscious although many of its functions occur without conscious knowledge. The ego fulfils its executive function negotiating the demands of the id, the superego and external reality. It functions at all three conscious, preconscious and unconscious levels adapting through use of defences. The ego ideal is that part of the developing ego that is allocated the function of preserving mental parental images.

3 Superego This is the censor of the personality. It is the individual's morals, values and ethics as derived from his/her parents. Its conscious component is termed conscience. An individual is aware of their morality but not the processes that operate to generate or sustain it. The superego develops in the second year of life and is established by the age of 5 years.

Psychotherapy and the psychotherapeutic relationship

Freud initially used the technique of **hypnosis** to recall suppressed memories. However, it was often unsuccessful and Freud believed that it hindered the free flow of thoughts. He therefore developed the **concentration method,** which requires the patient to lie down, close their eyes and concentrate on their symptoms. Freud would facilitate the process by the use of leading questions and by placing his hands on the patient's forehead. This was used to recall memories associated with the symptoms. From this Freud progressed to **free association** in which again the patient is lying down but with open eyes. The patient is then asked to voice any and all their thoughts as they arise without reservation or censorship.

Transference This unconscious process involves the displacement of feelings for significant others, usually family members, onto the therapist.

Countertransference The conscious feelings, emotions and attitudes of the therapist towards the patient.

Resistance Obstruction of access to the unconscious.

Psychosexual development

Freud proposed that psychosexual development took place in stages: (oral and anal phases collectively referred to as:

Pregenital/narcissistic phase (NB ages double, i.e. 1½, 3, 6 and 12 years.)

- 0–18 months   **Oral phase:** pleasure is derived from oral activity and there is a preoccupation with feeding.
  Sucking stage: passive early oral phase (receptive phase)
  Biting stage: aggressive oral (sadistic phase).
- 18–36 months **Anal phase:** Attention is focused on excretory processes. Infant has to adapt to the demands of others.
  Expulsive and retentive phases.
- 3–6 years   **Phallic phase:** increasingly focus on genitalia and libido is directed towards others.
  Involves castration anxiety, penis envy, oedipal* complex in males and electra[†] complex in females (attachment to opposite sex parent and aggression towards same sex parent).
- 6–12 years   **Latency:** up till the onset of puberty. Involves the recognition, acknowledgement and acceptance of reality.

(*Oedipal complex: in Sophocles' tragedy Oedipus Rex kills his father and marries his mother, not knowing their true identities.

[†]Electra complex: from Greek mythology, Electra plans the death of her mother Clytemnestra, responsible for the murder of her father.)

Genital phase

- 12 years–adult   Acquisition of sexual maturity (narcissistic, homo-sexual and heterosexual experiences)

Freud's theories on dreams

In *The interpretation of dreams* Freud described dreams as the 'royal road to the unconscious'. He set out the composition of dreams and the basic principles for their interpretation:

- dreams aim to preserve sleep
- they consist of **latent** and **manifest** components
- dreams represent the fulfilment of **unconscious wishes**.

The latent dream is disguised and transformed into the manifest dream through dream work which consists of four mechanisms:

- dramatization/symbolization: symbols are used to represent abstract ideas
- displacement: latent content is replaced by obscurely related elements
- condensation: latent elements are fused and abbreviated
- secondary elaboration: the revision that occurs upon waking; rationalizing the dream.

Anna FREUD (1892–1982)

Daughter of Sigmund Freud. Along with others, elaborated upon defence mechanisms: *CUPIDS RAFT*

(NB defences can be categorized as narcissistic, neurotic, immature and mature.)

Compensation: attempts (conscious/unconscious) to make up for perceived deficiencies within oneself.

Undoing: (symbolic atonement) involves the negation of prior unacceptable behaviour. Counteraction is used to nullify the previous experience. Similar to reaction formation.

Projection: the attribution to another of unacceptable thoughts, motives and feelings that are actually one's own.

Projective identification: the association of unwanted, repressed and uncomfortable aspects of oneself with another through projection, resulting in identification.

Intellectualization: closely related to rationalization, this involves the excessive use of intellectual concepts and processes to avoid the expression of feelings. Affective experiences are thought about as opposed to being experienced.

Isolation: the separation of an idea from its attached original affect, breaking the links between the unacceptable impulse or act and its original memory and in so doing removing associated emotions.

Idealization: overestimation of an object's qualities.

Introjection: the transposition of external objects and their qualities into the self; the symbolic assimilation and internalization of an object. Central to the development of the ego and superego it is a form of identification, the opposite of projection.

Identification: the unconscious adoption of desirable attributes of others enhancing the individual's self-esteem through affiliation. It is important in the development of the superego.

Incorporation: thought to commence in the oral phase this is a special form of introjection that is central to the process of identification. It is a primitive defence that involves the assumption of another individual's characteristics.

Denial: the unconscious refusal to accept or acknowledge external reality.

Displacement: the transfer (redirection) of ideas and emotions concerning an object from this, the original, to a more acceptable or suitable substitute. Related to the process of symbolization.

Distortion: the remodelling and alteration of external reality to meet personal requirements or wishes.

Dissociation: unconscious detachment of particular mental processes from the remainder. This psychological separation leads to compartmentalization of functioning.

Suppression: this is the exclusion by volition of unacceptable ideas from the conscious. It is a conscious process (and hence by many not considered to be a true defence mechanism) that allows the impulse or conflict to be recalled.

Sublimation: the diversion of socially unacceptable instincts and drives into socially appropriate, creative activities.

Substitution: a highly valued but inconceivable goal or object is unconsciously supplanted by one that can be.

Symbolization: representation of objectionable ideas/objects with neutral ones through unconscious means. Results in the transfer/displacement of associated emotions to the symbol.

Somatization: the expression of psychological phenomena as bodily symptomatology. The preoccupation with somatic symptoms is disproportionate to physical findings.

Splitting: an inability to integrate opposing aspects of personality. Manifests as the polarized division of objects into good or bad.

Repression: most basic defence and most commonly employed. Unacceptable ideas, impulses or feelings are automatically shunned and banished into the unconscious.

Regression: unconscious retreat at times of stress to maturationally earlier level of emotional functioning. Lower level of complexity makes gratification more attainable.

Reaction formation: behaviour or attitude is directed such that it completely opposes the individual's underlying, unacceptable impulses. It involves two steps: the first is the repression of an unacceptable desire or wish and the second is the conscious expression of its direct opposite.

Rationalization: involves retrospective justification by way of offering rational, logical or acceptable explanations for ideas, feelings or behaviours that have unrecognized unworthy motives. It is a common unconscious defence and as such differs from lying which is a conscious process.

Reversal: an instinct which, though maintaining its aim, is reversed in its choice of object.

Restitution: the replacement of a lost, highly valued object by another.

Acting out: the expression of unconscious emotional difficulties as actions without conscious awareness of their significance.

Fixation: excessive gratification at an immature level of development because of the cessation of maturation.

Fantasy: daydreaming, that is, the creation or fabrication of mental images of events. Often an escape from reality allowing the fulfilment of wishes.

Turning against the self: impulses or aggression directed at others are turned against oneself.

Carl Gustav JUNG (1875–1961)

Born in Kesswil, Switzerland; only child until the age of 9.

Member of Freud's group and influenced by works of Immanuel Kant, Friedrich Nietzsche, Emmanuel Swedenborg and Richard von Kraft-Ebing.

Founder of analytical psychology.

Essential elements of Jungian theories:

The unconscious

In addition to the **personal unconscious,** Jung proposed a **collective unconscious** also called the **objective psyche,** which consists of autochthonous ideas and primordial images. He suggested that these universal memories of mankind contain inherited primitive cultural and racial elements which give rise to consciousness. The personal unconscious is relatively superficial and more accessible.

The libido

Jungian theory places less emphasis on the sexual role of the libido. The libido stems from all psychic and life energy. This psychic energy has two basic attitudes. **Introversion** is an inwardly directed libido manifest as self-preoccupation, and **extroversion** is an outwardly directed libido.

Psychological functions

Four basic operations of the mind: *FIST*

*F*eelings
*I*ntuition
*S*ensations
*T*hinking

Combination of the two attitudes (introversion/extroversion) and four functions creates eight psychological types (e.g. extrovert feeling, introvert feeling and so on).

Archetypes

Contents of the collective unconscious, numinous and primordial. **Archetypal images** (symbols): universal, symbolic images and related instinctual processes featured in dreams and myths

- **Persona** (mask portraying mood in Greek drama): 'social mask' enveloping the personality. Allows individual to conform to social expectation whilst satisfying personal needs. That part of consciousness that interacts and negotiates with external reality.
- **Soul-image** (anima and animus): paired with persona, it is its unconscious counterpart. **Animus**, male prototypical archetype; the male component of female personality. **Anima**, female prototypical archetype; the female component of male personality.
- **Shadow**: paired with the ego the shadow is its unconscious counterpart comprising repressed inferior or primitive animal instincts.
- **Self:** develops as individual deals with other archetypes binding together conscious and unconscious elements. It is the goal that individuation wishes to achieve, i.e. a complete, whole personality.
- **Complexes:** networks of ideas and thoughts linked through commonality of emotions and feelings. Surround archetypes and evolve out of archetype–experience interactions.
- **Individuation:** growth of an individual's personality leading to self-realization and understanding.

Jung's ideas have been criticized for being too mystical and difficult to test.

Melanie KLEIN (1882–1960)

Born in Vienna, the youngest of four. Became an important influence in the British Psycho-Analytical Society.

Important aspects of Kleinian theory:

Object relations theory

Infant capable of object relations and internalizes experiences of the external world.

Paranoid–schizoid position

Develops in first year of life and features sense of persecution and isolation. Infant uses defences of splitting, projective identification and introjection in dealing with the world and its environment. Frustration and anxiety are seen as necessary for the development and growth of the infant's personality. Good objects or part objects are internalized (introjected) whilst bad objects or part objects are projected.

Depressive position

Commences as infant begins to recognize its mother (age 6 months) and realizes the imperfections of the world. Begins to view objects as a whole and not as part objects and reconciles good and bad component of mother as one. Anxiety is transformed from paranoid to depressive form. Infant recognizes that it is separate from mother and that its **aggression** has been instrumental in this separation.

Alfred ADLER (1870–1937)

Viennese doctor. Founder of **individual psychology** (each individual achieves their particular personal goals in their own unique manner).

Important concepts:

Organ inferiority

Individuals have a desire for superiority, through self-improvement, and seek a particular lifestyle. This relates to their need for others and a desire for a sense of belonging. At birth the individual starts in an inferior position which causes anxiety and so the individual attempts to overcome this. The conscious and unconscious conflict that drives an individual to strive to overcome their anxiety is described as their **inferiority complex** (particularly when their desire or attempts at self-improvement are blocked or fail). Neuroses are then dysfunctional means by which individuals deal with their inferiority.

In Adlerian theory individuals are able to direct their fate as opposed to being subject to unconscious drives. Creativity and social cooperation are essential, primary qualities of human beings.

Adler described **masculine protest** as an individual's attempt to escape a submissive, feminine role.

Adolf MEYER (1866–1950)

Founded **psychobiology**. Comprehensive and pluralistic approach to understanding psychological illnesses. Brought together biological and psychosocial aspects. **Holistic approach**.

Aimed to understand people and their illnesses in simplest terms possible (common-sense psychiatry).

Karen HORNEY (1885–1952)

Developed **holistic psychology**. Stressed the principle of **basic anxiety.**

Child could cope with the environment by moving:

- towards people: (compliant person)
- against people: (aggressive person)
- away from people: (detached person).

Horney's concept of the self:

- **actual self**
- **real self**
- **idealized self**.

Therapy involved: self-actualization, self-realization and dealing with the here and now.

Harry Stack SULLIVAN (1892–1949)

Proposed **interpersonal theory** of personality; i.e. interpersonal experiences form basis of personality development.

Donald WINNICOTT (1897–1971)

Psychoanalyst who initially trained as a paediatrician.

Studied the mother–baby relationship and formulated concepts:

- **good-enough mother:** responsive to baby's needs, adequately meeting these by balancing frustration and gratification. Through good parenting child gains autonomy and develops **capacity to be alone**.

- **pathological mother:** gives personal needs priority. Baby creates a **false self** so as to protect **true self**.

Object relations

Between ages of 4 and 18 months infant selects an object (**transitional object**) such as a toy or piece of clothing that it uses to allay its own anxiety. Assists in separation-individuation.

Karl ABRAHAM (1877–1925)

Student of Sigmund Freud. Expanded upon Freud's psychosexual stages of development. Subdivided some stages further into phases:

- oral stage → biting and sucking phases
- anal stage → anal–sadistic (destructive–expulsive) and anal–erotic (mastering-retentive) phases

Gordon ALLPORT (1897–1967)

Founder of **humanistic school** of psychology.

Individual strives to develop self-identity. Selfhood is achieved in stages.

Eric BERNE (1910–1970)

Developed **transactional analysis**.

Described individuals as having three ego states: the **Child** (childhood primitive elements), the **Adult** (the personality component that is able to appraise reality objectively) and the **Parent** (the component that represents the values of the parents of the individual). Used the term psychological **games** to describe the interaction between states.

Wilfred BION (1897–1979)

Applied the ideas of psychoanalysis to groups and described the three **basic assumptions**: pairing, fight–flight and dependency.

Summary of other important figures

Table 7.2   Major contributions to psychotherapy and psychology

Important figure	Contributions to psychotherapy and psychology
Otto RANK (1884–1939)	Anxiety stems from birth trauma. Primal anxiety
Sandor FERENCZI (1873–1933)	Active therapy and forced fantasies
Carl ROGERS (1902–1987)	Client-centred psychotherapy, unconditional positive regard
Heinz KOHUT (1913–1981)	Founded school of self-psychology
Jacob MORENO (1882–)	Psychodrama
Frederich PERLS (1893–1970)	Gestalt Therapy
Eric BERNE (1910–1970)	Developed transactional analysis
Wilhelm REICH (1897–1951)	Character defences 'armour'. Character types: hysterical, narcissistic, masochistic, compulsive
Sandor RADO (1890–1972)	Adaptational psychodynamics
Erich FROMM (1900–1980)	Types of personality: marketing, hoarding, receptive, exploitative, productive
Abraham MASLOW (1908–1970)	Self-actualization

Table 7.3   Important developments in therapy

Important figure	Therapy/treatment developed
FRANKL	Existential logotherapy
ELLIS	Rational Emotive Therapy
JANOV	Primal Therapy
ASSAGIOLI	Psychosynthesis
WOLPE	Systematic desensitization
MONIZ	Psychosurgery
SAKEL	Insulin Coma Therapy
CHARPENTIER	Chlorpromazine
CADE	Lithium
KUHN	Imipramine
CERLETTI and BINI	Electroconvulsive Therapy (ECT)
FOUIKES	Group Therapy

Table 7.4   Noted associations of some important figures

Important figure	Noted association
BEARD	Neurasthenia
BRIQUET	Hysteria
BRAID	Neurohypnotism
CHARCOT	Hysteria/hypnosis
CULLEN	Neurosis
DURKHEIM	Anomie
ESQUIROL	Hallucinations
FALRET	La folie circulaire
GREISINGER	Neuropsychiatry
HECKER	Hebephrenia
HULL	Hypnosis
JANET	Hysteria/psychasthenia
MAXWELL	Therapeutic community
KAHLBAUM	Catatonia
LANGFELDT	Schizophreniform psychosis
MAY	Anxiety
MESMER	Hypnosis (animal magnetism)
MOREL	Demence precoce
SCHNEIDER	First rank symptoms
SHELDON	Body types
STAHL	Animism
SZASZ	Myth of mental illness
WATSON	Behaviourism

⑧ Psychopathology

The study of abnormal states of mind can be based upon experiment (experimental), experience (phenomenological) or explanation of this (psychodynamic). Individual symptoms can be indicative of illness because of their severity or duration; however, it is usually the collective grouping of symptoms to form characteristic syndromes that provides the basis of diagnoses. Symptoms are often described as being primary or secondary both in terms of aetiology and occurrence. Temporally, primary symptoms are those that occur first and secondary symptoms are those that follow. In terms of causation, primary symptoms are direct products of the disease process whereas secondary symptoms are consequent upon these or arise because of a reaction to the primary symptoms or the disease process.

Disorders of speech, language and thought

- **Agrammatism:** syntax of speech is lost such that it is meaningless, even though fluency does not seem to be as impaired.
- **Akataphasia:** used by Kraepelin to describe thought disorder manifest in speech.
- **Alogia:** 'Poverty of speech'; limited and often restricted to single word responses to questions or prompts.
- **Aphasia:** central language difficulty results in an inability to emit, understand or repeat words. More often used is dysphasia; difficulty in doing the same.
- **Asyndesis†:** a lack of sufficient connections between successive elements of thought.
- **Autism:** fantasy directed thought characteristic of schizophrenia and schizoid personality (Bleuler) (normal thought considered to be reality directed).
- **Circumstantiality:** tendency to dwell upon minutia and unnecessarily incorporate irrelevancies into conversation and thought prior to eventually achieving the desired goal.
- **Clang association:** a syllable from one word is associated with another from a different word by virtue of its sound.
- **Concrete thinking:** unable to entertain abstract thoughts.
- **Derailment (Entgleisen)†:** main theme of thought is displaced by intrusion of subsidiary themes and then these too undergo displacement.
- **Desultory*:** thought in which ideas suddenly force their way into speech, out of context, whilst maintaining syntax and grammar.

- **Drivelling*:** components of a thought are complete but mixed up and muddled (muddling – Faseln), losing all organization and expressed in speech as drivelling.
- **Dysphonia:** impaired ability to vocalize.
- **Dysarthria:** articulation difficulty because of motor disorder.
- **Echolalia:** automatic and pointless imitation and repetition of another individual's speech or words.
- **Echologia:** repetition of another individual's speech using own words or phrases (i.e. not exact as in echolalia).
- **Fusion (Verschmelzung)*:** interweaving (fusion) of two differing streams or elements of thought.
- **Interpenetration†:** separate themes of thought permeate each other becoming reciprocally pervasive.
- **Logoclonia:** repetition of the last word's last syllable. Form of perseveration.
- **Logorrhoea:** voluble, garrulous, fluent speech. Pressure of speech.
- **Loosening of associations (formal thought disorder):** Bleuler used this term to describe the lack of connections in thought and considered this to be the central feature of schizophrenic thought disorder.
- **Malapropism:** ludicrous misuse of words.
- **Metonym†:** imprecise expression that only approximates to intended word or phrase.
- **Mutism:** complete loss of speech (consciousness unimpaired). Can occur in schizophrenia, depression and organic brain disorders. Elective mutism is observed in children who choose to remain mute in certain instances/situations (often at school).
- **Neologism:** new word or novel use of a familiar word.
- **Obsessions:** senseless, repetitive, intrusive thoughts recognized by the individual as being irrational, who whilst acknowledging the thoughts as their own attempts unsuccessfully to resist them. They are rarely acted upon and usually concern; sex, contamination, aggression and religion.
- **Omission*:** senseless omission of a segment of thought.
- **Overinclusion†:** an inability to circumscribe a problem or retain meaningful boundaries.
- **Palilalia:** repetition of a word with increasing frequency. Usually the last word of a phrase or sentence.
- **Paralogia:** the verbal expression of positive thought disorder, because of difficulty in logical thought and reasoning.
- **Paragrammatism:** comprehensible phrases that collectively fail to make sense or convey any meaning.
- **Paraphasia:** substitution of a word or phrase with one that is wrong or distorted in some manner. Can be described as verbal or literal paraphasia. Can also be described as phonemic, resulting in mispronunciation or semantic producing malapropism.

- **Perseveration:** persistence of cued speech beyond its relevance.
- **Phobia:** persistent irrational fear that cannot be extinguished with reasoning despite awareness of its irrationality leading to avoidance. The fear is disproportionate to any real threat and is not under voluntary control. Many types of phobias, e.g. agoraphobia, claustrophobia and social phobia.
- **Pressure of speech:** increased rate and quantity. Speech is rapid and difficult to interrupt.
- **Prolixity:** flight of ideas in which the train of thought eventually returns to its original track.
- **Schizophasia (word salad, speech confusion):** words are jumbled up such that speech is difficult to understand.
- **Stammering:** pauses or the repetition of word fragments interrupt the normal flow of speech. Stammering may be accompanied by grimacing and is more marked when anxious. Also referred to as **stuttering**.
- **Stock word:** one which is used in a peculiar manner to have more than its usual significance or meaning.
- **Substitution*:** a principal thought or idea is replaced by a subsidiary thought or idea.
- **Tangentiality:** oblique verbal response, glancing at gist.
- **Thought block (snapping off; Entgleiten):** inexplicable, unanticipated, abrupt cessation of thought.
- **Verbigeration:** repetition of fragmented phrases in a form of verbal stereotyping.
- **Vorbeireden:** talking 'past the point' or **Vorbeigehen:** used by Ganser to describe 'passing by the point' or the 'approximate answer'. Responses to questions although incorrect betray comprehension.

* part of classification of thought disorder proposed by Schneider.

† part of classification of thought disorder proposed by Cameron.

Disorders of emotion

- **Affect:** short-lived observable pattern of behaviour that expresses the subjective emotional state of an individual. It is subject to variation over brief periods of time.
- **Alexithymia:** inability to verbally express one's emotions.
- **Anhedonia:** subjective inability to gain enjoyment or pleasure from activities that would normally provide gratification.
- **Anosodiaphoria:** emotional indifference to disease.
- **Anxiety:** a feeling of intense inner tension, apprehension and fear, occasionally accompanied by somatic symptoms, experienced in the context of an anticipated threat.

- **Apathy:** a complete loss of interest.
- **Asthenic affects:** horror, anxiety, grief, sadness and shame.
- **Belle indifference:** dissociation of affect in which the individual displays apparent detachment from their malady.
- **Blunting of affect:** emotional responsiveness is diminished.
- **Depression:** pervasive low mood that is sustained and qualitatively different from normality.
- **Dysphoria:** unpleasant mood.
- **Dysthymia:** chronic state of low mood, usually with an insidious onset and lasting at least two years.
- **Elation:** an elevation of mood or affect.
- **Euphoria** and **ecstasy:** describe happy and pleasant moods when within normal limits but in pathological states signify extreme cheerfulness and feelings of well-being.
- **Euthymia:** happy contented mood.
- **Flattening of affect:** emotional responsiveness is reduced to the extent that there is almost no evidence of affect or affective change.
- **Incongruity of affect or mood:** dissonance between an individual's mood and their circumstances or topic of conversation.
- **Lability of mood:** rapidly changing emotions. Mood tends to fluctuate with unusual rapidity. Extreme lability of mood with total loss of emotional control is described as **emotional incontinence**.
- **Mood:** sustained and pervasive emotion. (NB clinically, the terms affect and mood are often used interchangeably.)
- **Moria (fatuous affect): Witzelsucht;** apathy and silliness combined with general indifference.
- **Perplexity:** anxiety and puzzlement.
- **Sthenic affects:** hate, anger, rage and joy.
- **Verstimmung:** ill-humoured mood state (moodiness) usually with depressive symptoms which via the individual's behaviour 'spills out' onto surrounding others making them unhappy as well.

Disorders of belief

Overvalued idea An intense, sustained, unreasonable preoccupation that is held with less than delusional conviction. It represents beliefs that are between delusional and non-delusional. The individual accepts the possibility of their belief being erroneous and the belief itself is usually not one that is held by others from a similar background.

Delusion A fixed, false belief that is not in keeping with the individual's cultural background or the beliefs of their peers. An abnormal belief of morbid origin. Delusional themes:

Delusions of:

- guilt and worthlessness
- ill-health (Cotard's syndrome)
- persecution (querulant delusions; paranoid delusions)
- reference
- grandeur
- love (erotomania; de Clerambault's syndrome)
- jealousy (morbid jealousy; Othello syndrome)
- poverty
- infestation (Ekbom's syndrome)
- religion

Autochthonous delusion (primary delusion) A well-formed delusion that appears suddenly without any apparent connection with past or ongoing matters. Often follow a period of 'delusional mood'.

Delusional mood (Wahnstimmung) A period of uncertainty during which the individual 'senses' or feels that something of significance is about to take place.

Nihilistic delusion Delusional belief of negation and nothingness. Nothing exists; mind, body, world. Occurs in Cotard's syndrome. Occasionally associated with delusions of enormity.

Passivity phenomena (delusions of control) Individual believes that an outside agency is able to control and influence their actions, impulses and thoughts, processes that are normally under their own control.

- 'made' feelings, impulses and actions
- somatic passivity
- thought insertion: individual believes that their thoughts are introduced by an external agency: Cf. obsessional thoughts, recognized as own.
- thought withdrawal: individual believes that their thoughts are removed by an external agency (often able to describe sensation of thoughts leaving)
- thought broadcast: individual believes that their thoughts are shared with others by virtue of them being 'broadcast' by some means (radio, television, telepathy)

Delusional perception (apophanous perception)

Novel delusional interpretation of a normal perception which cannot be completely understood in terms of the patient's mental state. The latter component differentiates delusional perception from delusional misinterpretation.

Delusional misinterpretation

Individual attaches delusional meaning to a normal perception in the context of a pre-existing delusion.

Delusional misidentification

Consists of four related syndromes:

- **Capgras syndrome** (l'illusion de sosies): individual believes that a closely related or familiar person has been supplanted by an impostor who is an exact double. In specific case of where spouse is thought to have been replaced this has been described as the 'Amphitryon illusion'. The belief that other people in addition to the spouse are doubles has been termed the 'Sosias illusion'.
- **Syndrome of Fregoli:** familiar person is falsely identified in complete strangers (reciprocal of Capgras).
- **Intermetamorphosis:** the exchange of individuals is reciprocal and those that are involved posses physical similarities in addition to psychological ones.
- **Subjective doubles** (doubles of the self): individual believes and maintains that another individual has been transformed into his own self.

Disorders of perception

Sensory distortions

Sensory apparatus is unchanged. Threshold and subsequent subjective experience of a percept are altered:

- Hyper- and hypo-acusis: changes in sensitivity to sound.
- Macro- (megalo-) and micro-psia: visual changes with respect to size.

False perceptions

Illusion False perception of a real stimulus (external). Three types:

- completion illusion
- affect illusion
- pareidolia: vivid, effortless illusion heightened in intensity with focusing of attention. (NB affect and completion illusions are extinguished by attention.)

Eidetic image Recollection of a memory as an hallucination; reproducing a vivid perception (common amongst children).

Hallucination Spontaneous, false perception occurring in objective space with the full force of a real perception in the absence of a real stimulus or object.

Auditory hallucinations

- elementary hallucinations; basic sounds, noises, whistles
- hearing voices (phonemes – Wernicke)
- own thoughts spoken aloud (Gedankenlautwerden – thoughts and voice are synchronous; Echo de la pensées – voice is heard immediately after thought). Alternative terms: thought echo and thought sonorization
- command hallucinations and imperative hallucinations
- running commentary and second or third person hallucinatory voices.

Somatic hallucinations

- superficial: involving sensations from skin, e.g. touch (haptic), temperature (thermic); NB formication (sensation of insects crawling on, in or beneath the skin)
- visceral: involving deep, inner sensations from viscera.

Olfactory and gustatory hallucinations

- may be prolonged, mood congruent and suggest temporal lobe epilepsy.

Visual hallucinations

- **Lilliputian hallucinations** (associated with alcohol withdrawal; often pleasurable)
- **autoscopic hallucination** (phantom mirror image; Doppelganger): visual hallucination of oneself

- **negative autoscopy:** upon reflection of oneself in a mirror no image is seen
- **experiential hallucinations:** visual hallucinations occurring in temporal lobe epilepsy (thought to be vivid memories).

Extracampine hallucinations Perceived outside of individual's field of perception.

Hypnogogic hallucinations Occur whilst *go*ing to sleep.

Hypnopompic hallucinations Occur whilst waking from sleep.

Functional hallucinations Both the normal percept and the hallucination that it produces are simultaneously perceived (NB the latter is not a modification of the former).

Reduplicative hallucinations Experience of an additional limb or body part (NB differs phantom limb in which the body part that is experienced has been lost).

Pseudohallucination Differs from normal perception and hallucination in that it is located in inner subjective space, it is not real and lacks tangibility/substantiality, it has the qualities of an idea and is therefore dependent upon the observer for its existence and can only do so in a specific modality.

Palinacousis Ictal phenomenon in which there is perseveration of an auditory sensation.

Phosphenes Flashes of light perceived upon direct stimulation of the occipital cortex.

Synaesthesiae Perceptions occurring in one sensory modality upon stimulation in another. When the perception is a hallucination it is described as **reflex hallucination**.

Disorders of movement

Adaptive movements

Expressive In general these involve the face and limbs. They are influenced by cultural norms and the emotional state of individual.

Catatonia Movements markedly diminished, and performed with stiff awkwardness. Expressionless face, mask-like. Characteristic of schizophrenia but is also seen in Parkinson's disease.

Omega sign and crow's foot Characteristic furrowing of the brow in depression.

Goal-directed Voluntary movements are usually performed effortlessly.

Obstruction (blocking) Central disorder resulting in irregular hindrance of motor activity. Often react at the last moment.

Psychomotor retardation Thoughts and actions are subjectively slowed with particular difficulty in initiation.

Mannerisms Repetitive, spontaneous, complex movements that were once purposeful.

Non-adaptive movements

Spontaneous movements

Tic(s) Sudden involuntary repetitive movement of a group of muscles.

Static tremor Occurs at rest, usually involving upper body parts, and is exacerbated by anxiety. Often familial, worsening with age, but can also be indicative of illness (Parkinson's disease, hyperthyroidism) or toxicity (lithium, alcohol). (Cf. intention tremor of cerebellar disease.)

Chorea Abrupt, jerking movements involving varying groups of muscles. Individuals with Huntington's chorea may attempt to hide the movements as habits.

Athetosis Serpentine, writhing movements, involving particularly the limbs distally and facial muscles. Absent in sleep.

Stereotypy Spontaneous, repetitive, possibly once purposeful movements that are not goal-directed and are socially unacceptable.

Induced movements

Echopraxia Automatic imitation of another individual's movements.

Perseveration Persistence of a cued movement beyond its relevance or appropriateness (stimulus has been withdrawn).

Automatic obedience (command automatism) Individual behaves in any manner that is requested regardless of any consequences.

Forced grasping Individual repeatedly grasps and shakes the offered hand despite instructions to the contrary.

Mitmachen (cooperation) A form of automatic obedience in which the individual, despite being requested to resist, allows their body to be freely positioned. However, upon release, body parts return to resting position.

Mitgehen A more extreme form of Mitmachen, in which even the slightest pressure initiates movement.

Opposition (Gegenhalten) Individual tries to oppose movements using a similar degree of force to that being applied. Resistance is apparently without motive and when accentuated is also referred to as **negativism**.

Ambitendency Individual is unable to complete an action, repeatedly starting and stopping.

Disorders of posture

Manneristic posture Unusual habitual postures that are exaggerations of the normal.

Perseveration of posture Individual briefly maintains any awkward posture in which they are positioned and then slowly relaxes. Plastic resistance against initial movement is called waxy flexibility (flexibilitas cerea).

Neuroanatomy, neurology and neuropathology

Neuroanatomy

Cellular components of the nervous system

The human nervous system consists of specialized cells called **neurones** (the functional units) and supporting cells called **neuroglia**.

Neurones Respond to stimuli with an electrical impulse that can be conducted over long distances.

Neurones have a cell body (**soma** or **perikaryon**) from which extend long processes in varying number. The latter can be an **axon,** of which there is usually one or many **dendrites**.

Axon (neurite; nerve fibre) Stems from soma as **axon hillock** to become **initial segment**. These parts of the axon are devoid of intracellular inclusions such as Nissl granules (ribosomes) and it is from here that the **axolemma** commences. Axons vary in length and can be myelinated or not. Terminal enlargements form synaptic boutons. A single neurone may form up to 10 000 synaptic connections with as many as 1000 neurones. Sympathetic and parasympathetic axons terminate in thousands of **synaptic varicosities**. Axons convey information away from the cell body.

Dendrite Receives information from other cells through thousands of receptor contacts and has **spines** (12 µm diameter) that increase the cell surface area and are the sites of synaptic connection. Dendrites convey information towards the cell body.

Axons and dendrites contain similar cytoskeletal components (microtubules, actin filaments and neurofilaments), however they differ significantly.

Nucleus Neuronal nuclei are spherical, central and 4–18 µm in diameter. Almost all neuronal nuclei have a **nucleolus** which is one-third their size and is necessary for protein synthesis.

Table 9.1   Comparison of axons and dendrites

Features	Axons	Dendrites
Morphology	Consistent diameter	Tapered
Arborization	Rare	Common
Conduction in relation to cell	Away	Towards
Numbers	Usually only one	Very many
Ribosomes	Nil	Yes
Cytoskeletal components	Neurofilaments > microtubules	Microtubules > neurofilaments
Specific proteins	Tau	MAP2

Classification Neurones can be described as **unipolar (pseudo-unipolar)** [dorsal root ganglion cells of peripheral nervous system and those in trigeminal mesencephalic nucleus], **bipolar** [some olfactory and retinal cells and those in acoustic ganglion (VIII)], or **multipolar** [spinal motor neurones, cerebellar Purkinje cells, cortical pyramidal cells, neurones of autonomic nervous system] depending upon the number of axons and dendrites they possess. Most CNS neurones are multipolar.

Alternatively, they can be described as **amacrine** (no axon), **Golgi type I** (long) or **Golgi type II** (short. 0.5–5 mm) according to axonal length.

Golgi type I neurones form commissures, tracts and association / projection fibres.

Golgi type II neurones remain within gray matter.

Neurones can also be described as afferent, efferent or interneurones.

- **Afferent neurones**: (sensory) mostly outside of CNS. Carry information towards spinal cord and brain.
- **Efferent neurones**: mostly outside of CNS. Autonomic efferents and motor neurones. Carry information to effector organs.
- **Interneurones**: originate and terminate within CNS. 99% of neurones are interneurones.

Neuroglia (glial cells/glia) First described by Virchow as nerve glue (neuro-glia). Glia make up 50% of brain volume and outnumber neurones 10:1. Unlike neurones, glia are non-conducting and continually undergo mitosis. They are separated from neurones by intercellular spaces and fulfil a variety of functions.

Types:

Astrocytes

- maintain chemical environment and take up excess K^+
- structural support of nervous tissue
- part of blood–brain barrier
- involved in phagocytosis and healing.

- **Protoplasmic astrocytes:** found mainly in grey matter, they have plenty of granular cytoplasm with a large nucleus and thick processes that flatten to form pedicles which adhere to neurones, blood vessels and pia mater.
- **Fibrous astrocytes**: predominantly in white matter, with longer but less branched extensions. Contain specific glial acidic fibrillary protein.

Oligodendrocytes

- less branches and are smaller than astrocytes
- stained by del Rio–Hortega's silver method
- have numerous ribosomes and mitochondria and an extensive rough endoplasmic reticulum and Golgi apparatus.
- synthesize myelin sheath (same as Schwann cells in peripheral nervous system)
- types:
  interfascicular: white matter
  perineuronal: grey matter
  perivascular: white and grey matter.

Microglia Derived from haematopoetic stem cells; small with elongated nuclei and a paucity of cytoplasm. Found more so in grey matter and from 10% of total glia. Proliferate following injury, inflammation or degeneration and hence likened to macrophages (both express receptors for Fc portion of immunoglobulins).

Ependyma Ciliated cells that line CNS cavities and aid CSF flow.

Types:

- ependymocytes (ventricles and spinal cord central canal)
- choroidal epithelial cells (cover choroidal plexi)
- tanycytes (floor of third ventricle overlying median eminence).

NB special kinds of glia in:

- retina: **Muller cells**
- posterior pituitary: **pituicytes**
- cerebellum: **Bergman cells**.

Nervous system development

3rd week of development – central nervous system (CNS) appears as **neural** or **medullary plate** (elongated thickened plate of ectoderm) occupying anterior portion of embryonic disk.

- Lateral edges fold to form **neural folds** and central neural groove.
- Neural folds fuse to form **neural tube** which separates from overlying ectoderm.
- Coinciding with this is mesodermal somite segmentation (muscles and axial skeleton).
- Neural tube closure commences at level of 4th somite and proceeds in both directions until anterior and posterior neuropores remain.
- **Anterior neuropore** closes day 25.
- Neural tube divides to form the brain and its components and the spinal cord.
- Cephalic portion of neural tube forms the three **primary brain vesicles**:
  - **Prosencephalon** (forebrain)
  - **Mesencephalon** (midbrain)
  - **Rhombencephalon** (hindbrain).

Differential rates of growth result in constrictions and flexions:

- cervical flexure (junction of hindbrain and spinal cord)
- cephalic flexure (midbrain)
- pontine flexure (separates metencephalon and myelencephalon). Flexion is opposite to cervical and cephalic flexion.

Table 9.2 Embryonic derivation of central nervous system structures

Embryonic structure	Adult derivative	Ventricular component
Telencephalon (forebrain)	Cerebral hemispheres (cortex) Hippocampus Basal ganglia Olfactory bulb	Lateral ventricles
Diencephalon	Hypothalamus Thalamus Subthalamus Epithalamus	III ventricle
Mesencephalon	Midbrain	Cerebral aqueduct (of Sylvius)
Metencephalon	Cerebellum and pons	IV ventricle
Myelencphalon	Medulla	IV ventricle
Spinal cord	Spinal cord	Central canal

(NB Alphabetical order of **mes**, **met**, **my**)

5th week of development:

- prosencephalon → telencephalon and diencephalon
- rhombencephalon → metencephalon and myelencephalon.

During gestation cortical neurones commence life cycle in close proximity to cerebral ventricles. Radial glial cells guide developing cortical neurones as they migrate (neuronal migration). Individual neurones stop migration at specific points and reach maturity developing dendritic and axonal connections.

Cerebral cortex (pallium)

Grey matter (lacks myelinated nerve fibres and blood vessels): variable thickness (1.5 mm calcarine fissure to 4.5 mm motor cortex), contains 15 billion neurones.

Telencephalon forms three layers:

- outer **marginal** layer – cerebral cortex
- intermediate **mantle:** – cerebral white matter
- inner **matrix** layer – surrounds lateral ventricles.

Cortical cell types

1 **Pyramidal**: most common, triangular cell bodies with apex pointing towards cortical surface. Vary in size 10–100 μm and found in all cortical layers except molecular layer. Giant cells (Betz) feature of precentral gyrus (motor area 4).
2 **Stellate** (Granule) cells: star-shaped and common with cell bodies of 4–8 μm. Present in all layers and greatest in layer IV.
3 **Fusiform** cells: usually spindle-shaped lying perpendicular to cortical surface and limited to deepest cortical layer.
4 **Horizontal cells of Cajal**: axis is parallel to cortical surface and are exclusive to molecular layer.
5 **Cells of Martinotti**: axon ascends from small cell body. Present throughout cortex but rare in molecular layer.

Cortical layers
Hippocampal formation (archipallium) and olfactory cortex (paleopallium) have three layers and are called allocortex. Neocortex (neopallium) forms 90% of cerebral cortex and consists of six layers:

I   Molecular layer: (plexiform layer) is outermost.
II   External granular layer: granular cells are Nissl stained rounded cell bodies of stellate cells.

III   External pyramidal layer: predominantly pyramidal cells.
IV   Internal granular layer: contains thalamic myelinated nerve fibres called external band of Baillarger.
V   Internal pyramidal layer: Betz cells in precentral motor cortex. Internal band of Baillarger.
VI   Fusiform layer: traversed by all fibres entering or exiting cortex.

Cortical maps

1905	Iain Campbell	20 areas	
1909	Korbinian Brodmann	52 areas	(Brodmann's areas (BA) still used)
1919	Cecile and Oscar Vogts	200+ areas	
1929	Constantinou von Economo	109 areas	

Cortex forms two convoluted hemispheres. Elevations are called **gyri**; depressions are called **sulci**. Deep sulci are called **fissures**. Each cerebral hemisphere consists of six lobes:

TO FLIP

Temporal
Occipital
Frontal
Limbic
Insular (central)
Parietal lobes

Temporal lobe Lateral aspect consists of three gyri (superior, middle, inferior) bounded by two sulci (superior, inferior). Superior aspect consists of transverse temporal gyri of Heschl (posterior part on left side forms Wernicke's area BA 22). Anterior aspect forms temporal pole and medial aspect consists of hippocampus, entorhinal cortex, amygdala and

Table 9.3 Temporal lobe lesions

Temporal lobe region	Effects of lesion
Medial	Anterograde amnesia L-side: verbal; R-side: non-verbal
Superior	L-side: Wernicke's sensory (receptive, fluent) aphasia; R-side: amusia
Posterolateral	L-side: semantic amnesia; R-side: prosopagnosia
Irritative lesion	Forced thinking, *déja vu, jamais vu*

parahippocampal gyrus. The uncus and adjoining parts of the para-hippocampal gyrus contain the olfactory receptive area which when damaged can lead to anomia. Irritative lesions can also cause uncinate fits (occasionally feature olfactory hallucinations as aura).

Additional manifestations of temporal lobe dysfunction:

- Upper homonymous quantrantanopia
- Non-dominant lobe: dysprosody
- bilateral: Korsakoff's amnesia, Kluver Bucy syndrome.

Occipital lobe Prominent calcarine sulcus on medial aspect.

Lobe contains primary visual cortex (BA 17) and association areas (BA 18 and 19).

Lesions inferior to calcarine fissure can lead to contralateral **hemichromatopsia**.

Additionally a L-sided lesion may cause dyslexia without agraphia.

Bilateral lesions superior to calcarine fissure can cause **Balint's syndrome**:

- optic ataxia (abnormal visual guidance of movements of limbs)
- oculomotor apraxia (inability to scan visual environment systematically)
- simultanagnosia (individual is unable to appreciate more than a single aspect of a stimulus configuration at any point in time; loss of panoramic vision; focus on central part of visual field).

Additional signs and symptoms of occipital lobe dysfunction; hallucina-tions and agnosias (prosopagnosia; visual agnosia; colour agnosia).

Frontal lobe (see also Chapter 3) Separated from parietal lobe by central sulcus (fissure of Rolando).

Consists largely of medial and lateral aspects.

Medial aspect divided into superior and inferior regions:

- superior region contains; anterior cingulate cortex and supplementary motor area
- inferior region contains; orbital cortex and basal forebrain.

Lateral aspect contains dorsolateral prefrontal cortex (DLPFCx) and frontal operculum which on dominant side contains **Broca's area** (BA 44 and 45).

Table 9.4 Frontal lobe lesions

Frontal lobe region	Effects of lesion
Superior medial aspect	Akinetic mutism
Orbital cortex	Personality changes: distribution, poor insight and judgement
Basal forebrain	Amnesia and confabulation
Dorsolateral prefrontal cortex	Impairment of cognitive and intellectual functions
Broca's area	Non-fluent, motor, expressive aphasia
Frontal operculum (non-dominant side)	Dysprosody
Irritative lesons	Eye deviation, amnesia

Limbic lobe Described by Willis as 'cerebri anatome' and by Broca (1878) as 'limbus' (border, ring) surrounding rostral brainstem and interhemispheric commissures. Lies beneath neocortex.

The limbic system can be defined according to development, function and connectivity hence some disagreement about constituents:

Limbic system:

- limbic cortex
- limbic nuclei
    subcortical
    associated.

Limbic cortex *COSH*

*C*ingulate gyrus	– overlying corpus callosum (CC) [BA 24,32]; allocortex
*O*lfactory (primary) cortex	– septal cortex
	– anterior perforated substance
	– prepyriform cortex (part of uncus of parahippocampal gyrus)
*S*eptal cortex	– septum pellucidum
(septal region below	– septal nuclei
CC genu)	– subcallosal gyrus
*H*ippocampal formation	

Subcortical limbic nuclei septal nuclei (beneath septal cortex)

- nucleus accumbens septi
- medial and lateral septal nuclei
- amygdala.

ABC

*A*mygdala
*B*asolateral amygdaloid (association with temporal lobe cortex)
*C*orticomedial amygdaloid

Associated limbic nuclei *MERIT*

*M*ammillary body hyopothalamic nuclei
*E*pithalamic habenular nucleus
*R*eticular formation of midbrain tegmentum
*I*nterpeduncular nucleus
*T*halamic anterior nucleus

Limbic system interconnections and circuits:

Amygdala — *stria terminalis* → **septal region** — *longitudinal striae* →
→ **dentate gyrus** → **hippocampus**

Amygdala ← *diagonal band* — **septal region** ← *fornix* — **hippocampus**

Limbic system receives inputs from all sensory systems.

Limbic system outputs are mainly from amygdala or hippocampus.

Papez circuit (main hippocampal output) links limbic system and neocortex via cingulate gyrus.

Hippocampus — *fornix* → **mamillary body** — *MTT* →
↑   → **ant. n. of thalamus** — *IC* → **cingulate gyrus**

multi-neuronal pathway

Amygdala output
|

stria medullaris
↓

habenular n. — *fasciculus retroflexus of Meynert* →
→ **interpeduncular n.** ⇒ **reticular formation**

Limbic system efferents:

- neocortex (conscious motor and sensory functions)
- hypothalamus (endocrine and autonomic function)
- brainstem reticular formation (arousal).

Limbic system lesions/stimulation effects:

Bilateral ablation of temporal lobe oral components (hippocampal formation, amygdala and uncus); causes **Kluver–Bucy syndrome**

VaPOrS

*V*isual *a*gnosia
*P*lacidity (loss of aggression/fear)
Hyper-*Or*ality (oral tendencies)
Hyper-*S*exuality (increased drive)

Limbic system lesions (especially mammillary body haemorrhage) cause failure of memory consolidation. Seen in Korsakoff's syndrome (poor anterograde memory).

Stimulation of:

- septal areas: diminishes aggression
- amygdala: promotes aggression and oral actions (biting, licking, swallowing).

Hippocampal formation

- hippocampus (Ammon's horn)
- dentate gyrus
- subicular complex (component of parahippocampal gyrus, PHG).

- **Hippocampus**: three principal layers.
    - **plexiform layer**: alveus (white matter) – contains pyramidal cell axons and afferent neurones and forms ventricular surface of hippocampal formation.
    - **pyramidal layer** – contains pyramidal cells
    - **polymorphic layer** – pyramidal cell main hippocampal cell; basket cells lie in proximity to pyramidal cells.

Stratum radiatum, lacunosum and moleculare are secondary laminae and comprise the **molecular layer**.

Stratum oriens consists of basket cells and basal dendrites.

Alveus axons form fimbria which form crura of fornix.

- **Parahippocampal gyrus** (PHG) (BA 28, enthorinal cortex): demarcated by collateral sulcus and continuous anteriorly with uncus, its superior aspect forms the subiculum. PHG has six-layer structure (neocortex). Subiculum along with hippocampal formation and dentate gyrus has three-layer structure (allocortex).
- **Dentate gyrus**: extends from indusium griseum to uncus between PHG and fimbria.
- **Indusium griseum:** (supracallosal gyrus, longitudinal striae): vestige of hippocampal formation.

Insular (central) lobe (island of Reil) Lies deep in **lateral (sylvian) fissure** and is circumscribed by circular sulcus.

Consists of long (posterior) and short (anterior) **oblique gyri** and a small medial projection to the anterior perforated substance called the **limen insula**.

Involved in autonomic functions and taste.

Substantia nigra (SN) Anatomically consists of two parts – pars compacta and pars reticulata. Pars compacta is darker (contains neuromelanin) and contains more neurones.

SN afferents: from

- striatum (the majority) (GABA)
- pallidum (GABA)
- nucleus coeruleus (NA)
- raphe nuclei (5-HT)
- subthalamic nucleus (glutamate).

SN efferents: to

- striatum
- thalamus
- superior colliculus
- reticular formation.

Parietal lobe The postcentral and intraparietal sulci divide the lobe into:

- Postcentral gyrus (sensory cortex) [BA 3,1,2]: somatotopic somatosensory area responsible for somesthesis (touch), vibration sense, kinesthesis (position) and epicritic touch (two-point discrimination).
- Posterior to postcentral gyrus are the superior and inferior parietal lobules (BA 7, part of 5 and 40); somatosensory association area involved in processing, realizing and storing sensory experiences.
- Supramarginal (BA 40) and angular gyrus (BA 39); components of inferior parietal lobule involved in reception and organization of language (particularly dominant hemisphere).
    - bilateral: astereognosia
                   agraphognosia
                   autotopagnosia
    - unilateral: dominant parietal lobe –
                   finger agnosia; alexia with agraphia +/- apraxia
                   right–left disorientation; pain asymbolia
                   ideomotor apraxia
                   non-dominant parietal lobe –
                   sensory inattention (neglect) i.e. anosognosia
                   dressing apraxia; constructional apraxia
                   geographic disorientation.

'Gerstmann's syndrome' (dominant parietal lobe):

- agraphia
- right–left disorientation
- finger agnosia
- aculculia
- alexia.

Table 9.5   Parietal lobe lesions

Parietal lobe region	Effects of lesion
Post central gyrus	Sensory loss
Optic radiation	Lower homonymous quadrantanopia
Non-dominant	Apraxia, anosognosia
Dominant	Gerstmann's syndrome
Inatative lesion	Somatic hallucinations

Basal ganglia (BG)

These subcortical telencephalic gray masses consist of neurones and intermingled axons.

The internal capsule separates the BG form the diencephalon. The BG are:

1 corpus striatum = caudate nucleus and = putamen (shell) and
                         lenticular (lentiform)   globus pallidus (pale
                         nucleus   globe)

2 amygdaloid nuclear complex (amygdala)
3 claustrum.

NB striatum (neostriatum) = caudate nucleus plus putamen (i.e. corpus striatum minus globus pallidus)

paleostriatum = pallidum = globus pallidus

BG connections and pathways

 – afferents to neostriatum
      cerebral cortex
      thalamus
 – afferents to globus pallidus
      neostriatum
      subthalamic nucleus
 – efferents from neostriatum
      globus pallidus and substantia nigra
 – efferents from globus pallidus
      subthalamus
      thalamus
      hypothalamus
      reticular formation
      substantia nigra.

Signs of basal ganglia lesions Origin of extrapyramidal tract which modulates motor activity and tone.

Extrapyramidal tract fibres act within central nervous system and on corticospinal tract and not on lower motor neurones or spinal cord.

Basal ganglia damage results in involuntary movement disorders:

  – parkinsonism, chorea, athetosis, hemiballismus.

Frontal-subcortical circuits

Parallel circuits connecting frontal cortex, BG and thalamus:

Table 9.6 Frontal-subcortical circuits

Circuit (modal)	Function
Motor	Motor
Oculomotor	Eye movements
Dorsolateral prefrontal	Cognition
Anterior cingulate	Motivation
Lateral orbitofrontal	Personality

Neurology

Cranial nerves

I Olfactory n. 1° neurones – nasal mucosa olfactory receptors communicate via cribriform plate of ethmoid bone.

2° neurones – olfactory bulb mitral cell axons pass to trigone via olfactory tract and lateral olfactory striae to reach primary olfactory area.

3° neurones – connect to olfactory association area. Anterior PHG (BA 28).

Anosmia: causes

  – common   head injury
               olfactory groove meningioma
  – rare   frontal lobe tumour
               obstructive hydrocephalus.

II Optic n. (see Figure 9.1)

  1 Retinal lesions: can cause scotomata or tunnel vision:
        tunnel vision: glaucoma
                         papilloedema
                         retinitis pigmentosa

SCOTOMA

Senile macular degeneration
Compression of nerve
Optic neuritis
Toxins (tobacco)
Olfactory groove meningioma
Malignancy (optic n. glioma)
Alcohol (thiamine deficiency)

2 Optic n. lesions: those of
scotoma and:
papilloedema
ischaemia
syphilis.

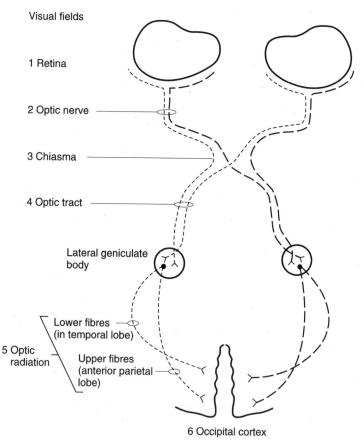

Figure 9.1 *Visual pathways*

3 Chiasma lesions: cause
    unilateral/bilateral temporal hemianopia
    *p*ituitary tumour (*u*pper fields affected first)
    craniopharyngioma (lower fields affected first)
    aneurysm.

4, 5 and 6 Lesions of optic tract, radiation and cortex cause
homonymous hemianopias and quadrantic defects (usually ischaemia
or tumours).

Optic tract lesions often lead to incongruous visual fields.

Optic radiation lesions do not show macular sparing and when causing
quadrantanopias; upper outer defect because of lesion in contralateral
anterior temporal lobe; lower outer defect-parietal lobe lesion.

*T*emporal – *T*op

Occipital cortex lesions show macular sparing because usually due to
post. cerebral artery infarction

*M*acular region supplied by *M*iddle cerebral artery

Eye reflexes (see Figure 9.2)

Light reflex:

Retina — *optic n.* → pretectal area — (crossed) →
    → Edinger Westphal nuclei — *III n.* → ciliary ganglion →
    → sphincter pupillae

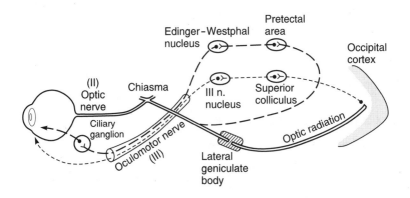

Accommodation reflex (- -): involves the cortex
Light reflex (—— ——): does not involve lateral geniculate body or cortex
Convergence originates in cortex and is relayed to pupils via III n. nuclei
and oculomotor nerves.
Relaying of consensual reflexes takes place at brainstem level

Figure 9.2 *Visual reflexes*

Accommodation reflex:

Retina — *optic n.* → **Lateral geniculate body (LGB)** —
— **optic radiation** → **cortex** → **superior colliculus** →
→ **III n. nucleus** — *III n.* → **eye muscles**

NB Ac*c*ommodation reflex is *c*ortical. Light reflex is brainstem based.

Pupils

Table 9.7 Pupil pathology

Pupil	Reaction to light	Causes
Small	Yes	Horner's syndrome, senile miosis
Small	No	Miotic drugs, opiates, Argyll Robertson, pontine haemorrhage
Large	Yes	Holmes–Adie, anxiety
Large	No	Mydriatic drugs, III n. palsy, midbrain haemorrhage, brain death

III Oculomotor nerve Two motor nuclei:

- somatic efferent n. – supplies ocular muscles other than lateral rectus and superior oblique
- Edinger–Westphal n. – parasympathetic supply to ciliary muscles and constrictor pupillae.

Lesions: paralysis of eyelid. Eye is deviated down and out. Pupil dilated with no response to light (physical cause). Normal pupil suggests PS fibres spared as in diabetes.

IV Trochlear nerve Supplies superior oblique.

Lesion: failure of downward gaze during adduction.

VI Abducens nerve Supplies lateral rectus.

Lesion: Commonest ocular palsy. Eye deviated towards nose.

Causes of III, IV and VI n. palsies: vascular, neoplasm, raised intracranial pressure, diabetes, multiple sclerosis, encephalitis.

V Trigeminal nerve Largest cranial nerve with four nuclei:

- mesencephalic nucleus (proprioception)
- main sensory nucleus (touch)
- spinal nucleus (pain and temperature)
- motor nucleus.

Sensory components Three sensory nuclei receive sensations via three main branches:

- ophthalmic n.: frontal, lacrimal and nasociliary n. branches supply:
  upper eyelid, anterior scalp, lacrimal gland, lateral conjunctiva, eyeball, nasal skin and mucosa
- maxillary n.: infraorbital, superior alveolar and zygomatic n. branches supply:
  upper teeth, cheek, roof of mouth and soft palate
- mandibular n.: auriculotemporal, buccal, inferior alveolar and lingual n. branches supply:
  skin of temple and cheek, lower lip, teeth and chin and anterior two-thirds of tongue.

Motor component Supplies:

- muscles of mastication (massesters and pterygoids)
- temporalis.

Reflexes:

Corneal reflex: earliest to be affected. Afferent of corneal touch is unilateral trigeminal (ophthalmic), efferent (bilateral blink) is bilateral facial n.

Jaw reflex: hyper-reflexia indicative of upper motor neurone lesion.

Glabbelar tap: blinking *p*ersists in *P*arkinson's.

Damage due to demyelination, injury, tumour, infection.

VII *Facial nerve* Principal nuclei that serve three main functions:

Sensory nucleus of tractus solitarius Receives taste sensation from anterior two-thirds of the tongue, hard and soft palate and floor of the mouth. Carried in chorda tympani (branch of VII n. that joins trigeminal lingual n.).

Parasymapathetic nucleus Secretomotor function for lacrimal, sublingual and submandibular other glands (test lacrimation with Shirmer's test).

Motor nucleus Motor supply to facial muscles. Test by asking for a smile, closure of eyes tightly and to look up.

Facial weakness Upper half of face has bilateral (additional contralateral) innervation. Therefore upper motor neurone lesion leads only to weakness of lower portion of face. Lower motor neurone lesion affects whole face. Common idiopathic cause (Bell's palsy).

Facial n. passes through facial canal in temporal bone, stylomastoid foramen and parotid gland. Branches of facial nerve: temporal, zygomatic, buccal, mandibular, cervical.

VIII Vestibulocochlear nerve Cochlear n. – responsible for hearing.

Vestibular n. – responsible for maintenance of balance/equilibrium.

Tests for deafness: using tuning fork. (512Hz)

Weber test Tuning fork stimulated and placed at vertex.

If hearing is normal sound appears to emanate mid-line.

Conduction deafness – sound louder in affected ear.

Nerve deafness – sound louder in normal ear.

Rinne test Normally air conduction is better than bone. Tuning fork stimulated and placed initially base upon mastoid bone and then fork is held in line with meatus. Air > Bone is normal Rinne-positive. If not then Rinne negative, i.e. conduction deafness.

Conductive deafness: wax, infection (otitis media).

Perceptive deafness:old age (presbyacusis), trauma, tumour, infection (mumps, rubella).

Inner ear or brainstem pathology can cause **vertigo** (unsteadiness with subjective sensation of rotation).

IX Glossopharyngeal nerve Has three major nuclei – motor, parasympathetic and sensory.

Plays role in sensory arc of **gag reflex.**

Also conducts taste from posterior one-third of the tongue.

X Vagus nerve Has three major nuclei – motor, parasympathetic and sensory.

Motor supply to larynx and pharynx. Motor component of **gag reflex.**

Test by asking patient to say 'Aah'; if damaged, uvula moves to intact side.

Parasympathetic component important in visceral functions of heart, lungs, gastrointestinal tract.

XI Spinal accessory nerve Cranial root: supplies larynx, pharynx and soft palate.

Spinal root: supplies trapezius and sternocleidomastoid muscles.

XII Hypoglossal nerve Supplies muscles of the tongue.

If nerve is damaged, upon protrusion tongue deviates to affected side.

Bulbar and *pseudobulbar* palsy Concern cranial nerves IX, X and XII.

Both lead to dysarthria and dysphagia.

Clinical distinction of u***pp***er motor neurone (UMN) and lower motor neurone (LMN) damage made on basis of signs (Table 9.8):

Table 9.8 Bulbar and pseudobulbar palsy

	LMN – bulbar	UMN – pseudobulbar
Speech	Nasal	
Tongue	Flaccid; fasciculation	Spastic; small for mouth
Jaw jerk	Normal or absent	Brisk
Emotions	Normal	Labile
Cause	Infections, syringobulbia	Stroke, demyelination

Spinal cord

40–45 cm in length. About 1 cm diameter. Extends from medulla oblongata to conus below which spinal nerve roots form cauda equina. Cervical and lumbar enlargements because of extra fibres for limbs.

31 spinal nerves emerge symmetrically either side of spinal cord and leave vertebral canal via intervertebral foramina. Each spinal nerve is formed from dorsal and ventral roots which unite within the intervertebral foramina to form the spinal ganglia. The 31 pairs of spinal nerves are grouped as follows (8 cervical; 12 thoracic; 5 lumbar; 5 sacral; 1 coccygeal).

Peripheral neuropathy

- Hypertrophic (p***ALPA***ble) neuropathy:

  Acromegaly
  Leprosy
  Peroneal muscular atrophy (Charcot–Marie–Tooth)
  Amyloidosis

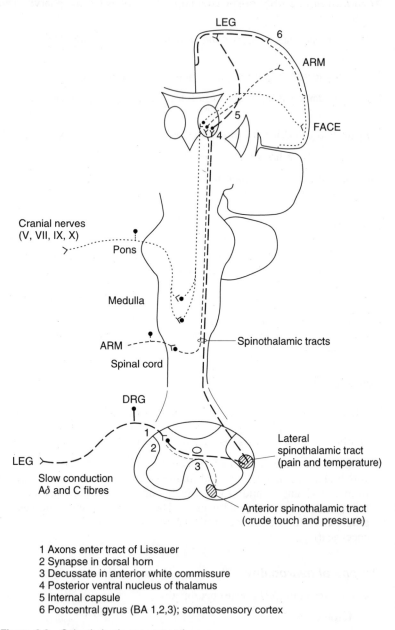

1 Axons enter tract of Lissauer
2 Synapse in dorsal horn
3 Decussate in anterior white commissure
4 Posterior ventral nucleus of thalamus
5 Internal capsule
6 Postcentral gyrus (BA 1,2,3); somatosensory cortex

Figure 9.3 *Spinothalamic sensory pathways*

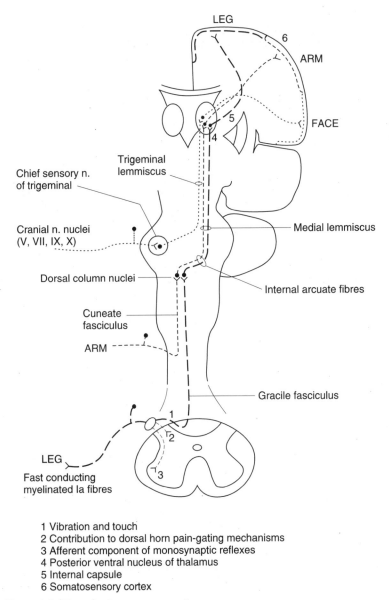

1 Vibration and touch
2 Contribution to dorsal horn pain-gating mechanisms
3 Afferent component of monosynaptic reflexes
4 Posterior ventral nucleus of thalamus
5 Internal capsule
6 Somatosensory cortex

Figure 9.4   *Dorsal column sensory pathways*

- Motor neuropathy (predominantly):
  - Guillan–Barre syndrome
  - lead poisoning
  - peroneal muscular atrophy
  - porphyria (acute intermittent)
  - diphtheria
  - herpes zoster.

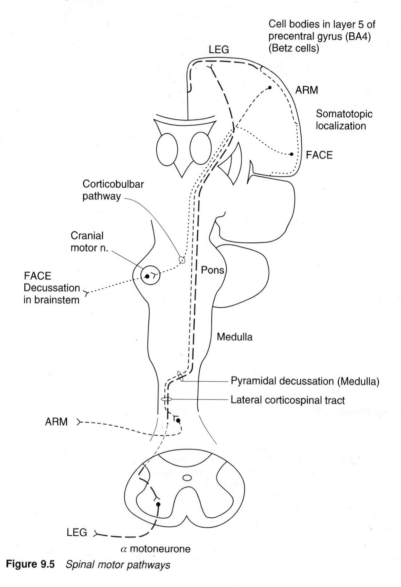

Figure 9.5 *Spinal motor pathways*

- Sensory neuropathy (predominantly):
  - nutritional deficiency (B12, folate)
  - amyloid
  - diabetes
  - uraemia
  - paraneoplastic.
- *PAIN*ful neuropathy:

  *P*oisoning (thallium)
  *AI*DS-related neuropathy
  *N*utritional

Blood supply of the brain

The brain receives blood from the internal carotid (branch of common carotid) and vertebral (branch of subclavian) arteries. The R and L vertebral arteries join at the level of the pons, ventral to the brainstem, to form the basilar artery. Branches from the basilar artery along with those from the internal carotid arteries form the circle of Willis at the base of the brain. The various branches and the parts of the brain they supply are shown in Figures 9.6 and 9.7.

If brain blood supply is compromised clinically it may lead to transient ischaemic attacks (TIAs) and cerebrovascular accidents (strokes). The signs and symptoms necessarily correspond to the parts of brain affected.

Carotid artery TIA symptoms and signs

- amaurosis fugax (ipsilateral)
- aphasia
- contralateral hemiparesis
- contralateral hemisensory loss
- retinal artery emboli.

Vertebrobasilar artery TIA symptoms and signs

- dysarthria
- dysphagia
- vertigo
- vomiting
- circumoral paraesthesiae
- drop attacks
- tinnitus
- transient global amnesia
- nystagmus
- ataxia.

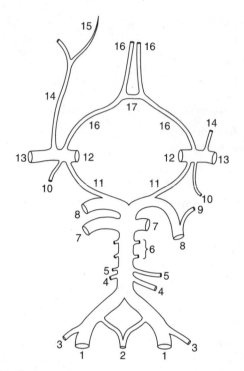

Figure 9.6 *Blood supply of the brain*

1 Vertebral
2 Anterior spinal
3 Posterior inferior cerebellar
4 Anterior inferior cerebellar
5 Labyrinthine (internal auditory)
6 Pontine
7 Superior cerebellar
8 Posterior cerebral
9 Posterior choroidal
10 Anterior choroidal
11 Posterior communicating
12 Internal carotid
13 Middle cerebral
14 Ophthalmic
15 Central retinal
16 Anterior cerebral
17 Anterior communicating

Anterior cerebral arteries Supply:

- medial aspects of orbital, frontal and parietal cortex
- anterior part of internal capsule
- basal nuclei.

Interruption may lead to:

- contralateral lower limb motor weakness and sensory loss
- incontinence
- release of primitive reflexes (palmo-mental, snout, grasp)
- akinetic mutism (bilateral frontal lobe damage).

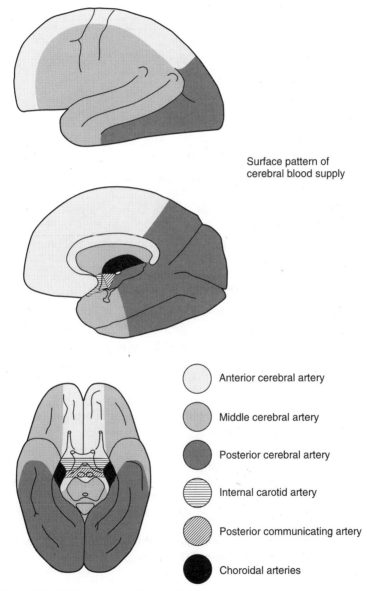

Surface pattern of
cerebral blood supply

◯ Anterior cerebral artery

◔ Middle cerebral artery

⬤ Posterior cerebral artery

▤ Internal carotid artery

▨ Posterior communicating artery

● Choroidal arteries

Figure 9.7   *Surface pattern of cerebral blood supply*

Middle cerebral arteries Supply:

- temporal, parietal and frontal cortex
- internal capsule
- basal nuclei.

Interruption may lead to:

- contralateral hemiplegia, hemianopia and sensory loss
- aphasia
- dressing apraxia
- contralateral neglect.

Posterior cerebral arteries Supply:

- inferior aspect of temporal and occipital (visual) cortex*
- posterior thalamus
- midbrain structures
- choroid plexus.

(*Macular area of visual cortex supplied by middle cerebral artery.)

Interruption may lead to:

- **midbrain (Weber's) syndrome**
    contralateral hemiplegia
    III nerve palsy
- thalamic syndromes
- homonymous hemianopia with macular sparing
- anomia.

Posterior inferior cerebellar artery (PICA) Occlusion leads to the **lateral medullary (Wallenberg's) syndrome**. It affects the brainstem and cerebellum and produces:

- Brain stem:
    - ipsilateral facial pain and temperature sensory loss*
    - laryngeal and pharyngeal (palatal) paresis because of damage to nucleus ambiguus
    - Horner's syndrome (ptosis and miosis) because of sympathetic fibre damage
    - contralateral limb and trunk pain and temperature sensory loss*
    (*together termed alternating hypalgesia).
- Cerebellum: *HAND*

    *H*ypotonia
    *A*taxia (ipsilateral limb) due to cerebellar tract damage
    *N*ystagmus
    *D*ysarthria

Basilar artery paramedian branch occlusion (penetrating mid-line branches) May result in a variety of syndromes:

- pontine level: Millard–Gubler syndrome
    abducens (VI cranial n.) and facial (VII cranial n.) palsy
    contralateral hemiplegia
- midbrain level: Benedikt's syndrome
    oculomotor (III cranial n.) palsy
    contralateral tremor (red nucleus – cerebellar output)
- medullary level: 'locked-in' (de-efferentation) syndrome (bilateral
    damage to anterior aspect of brainstem)
    complete bulbar palsy – hence mute
    interruption of corticospinal tracts leads to quadriplegia.

(NB retain ability to blink and move their eyes and are fully cognisant.)

Ventricular system

Consists of four communicating cavities within the brain. All are lined by
    ependyma and contain cerebrospinal fluid (CSF) produced from blood
    by the choroid plexuses within each ventricle.

There are two lateral ventricles (R and L) each communicating with a
    central third ventricle (III) via the interventricular foramen of Munro.

The third ventricle is connected to the ponto-medullary fourth ventricle
    (IV) via the cerebral aqueduct of Sylvius.

The fourth ventricle is continuous with the central canal of the spinal cord
    inferiorly and also communicates with the subarachnoid space via the
    *m*idline foramen of *M*agendie and the two *l*ateral foramina of *L*uschka
    (see Figure 9.8).

The choroid plexus is rich vascular tissue consisting of a network of pia
    mater blood vessels which project into each ventricle. Choroid plexus is
    covered by a layer of ependyma and secretes about 300–600 ml of CSF
    per day (NB ventricular volume is 25 ml and subarachnoid space volume
    is 110 ml). CSF is a colourless, clear, almost protein-free blood filtrate.
    It flows from the ventricles into the subarachnoid space and is eventually
    actively transported back into the blood circulation via superior sagittal
    sinus arachnoid granulations.

CSF pushes the arachnoid layer against the dura creating the subarachnoid
    space between the pia mater and the arachnoid. Its principal function is
    to support and protect the brain against trauma.

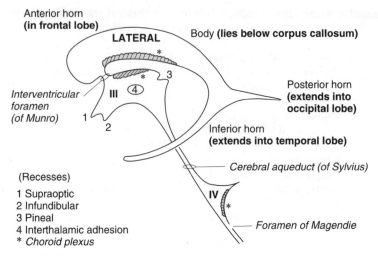

Anterior horn
(in frontal lobe)
LATERAL   Body **(lies below corpus callosum)**

Interventricular
foramen
(of Munro)

III   ④
3
1
2

Posterior horn
**(extends into
occipital lobe)**

Inferior horn
(extends into temporal lobe)

Cerebral aqueduct (of Sylvius)

(Recesses)
1 Supraoptic
2 Infundibular
3 Pineal
4 Interthalamic adhesion
* *Choroid plexus*

IV

Foramen of Magendie

Figure 9.8   *Ventricular system*

Hydrocephalus

1 Non-obstructive:	Communicating	e.g. brain atrophy (Alzheimer's disease)
2 Obstructive:	Communicating	e.g. Normal pressure hydrocephalus, meningitis, subarachnoid haemorrhage
3 Obstructive:	Non-communicating	e.g. obstruction of CSF flow within ventricular system, cerebral aqueduct stenosis, tumour.

Signs of cerebellar lesions

Single hemisphere damage leads to ipsilateral signs and usually intact hemisphere compensates for and eventually assumes lost functions.

- intention tremor (can be elicited with finger–nose or heel–shin test) with irregular rhythm (dysmetria)
- dysdiadochokinesia
- truncal ataxia
- ataxic gait
- dysarthria (scanning speech)
- hypotonia.

Disorders of gait

Cause	Gait
cerebellar	ataxia
normal pressure hydrocephalus	apraxia
Parkinson's disease	festinant gait
tabes dorsalis	steppage
stroke	hemiparetic gait (circumduction)

Tests of psychogenic signs and symptoms

Psychogenic blindness Eyes respond normally to spinning (vertically striped) cylindrical drum resulting in optokinetic nystagmus.

Psychogenic anosmia Usually individual claims a complete loss of smell. However, normally despite damage to the olfactory nerve (e.g. following head injury) the detection of noxious stimuli, e.g. ammonia, is retained through trigeminal innervation.

Psychogenic weakness 'Intermittent' as individual initially exerts some effort and then 'gives-way'. Can be demonstrated with the face–hand test (patient prevents their falling hand from hitting their face) or by eliciting Hoover's sign (individual inadvertently pushes 'weak leg' downwards whilst raising unaffected leg and fails to press down normal leg when lifting 'weak' leg).

Psychogenic gait impairment Astasia–abasia: individual staggers as if about to fall, grasping supports and people around them. In doing so they display balance, strength and coordination and do not usually fall.

Psychogenic sensory loss Distribution of loss does not correspond to anatomical patterns of sensory innervation. Midline demarcation of loss is exaggerated.

Psychogenic amnesia Individual claims of global loss of knowledge (including personal information), inability to acquire new information and scores less than predicted by chance on multi-choice recall.

Movement disorders

Parkinson's disease (PD) (James Parkinson 1755–1824)

Prevalence 1–2/1000 (1/200 age >70years).

Parkinsonism IDiOPATHIc

*I*diopathic (paralysis agitans) – commonest, insidious onset (age 50–60yr), with tremor often first sign. Progressive and initially asymmetrical presentation.

*D*rug induced – neuroleptics cause symmetrical slowness, rigidity and dystonic movements. Tremor less common.

*O*rganic disorders – 'Parkinsonism plus':progressive supranuclear palsy; primary autonomic failure (Shy–Drager syndrome), olivopontocerebellar degeneration, Huntington's disease, Creutzfeldt–Jakob disease.

*P*ost-encephalitic Parkinsonism – following encephalitis lethargica outbreaks (neurofibrillary changes are characteristic feature).

*A*therosclerosis – occurs in setting of vascular disease (ischaemia, hypertension, stroke) presents mainly with rigidity and bradykinesia (little tremor). Poor response to medication.

*T*rauma – dementia pugilistica.

*H*ydrocephalus (normal pressure).

*I*ntoxication – carbon monoxide, heavy metals, e.g. manganese, copper (Wilson's disease), MPTP (methyl phenyl tetrahydro pyridine – byproduct of illicit narcotic manufacture that specifically causes substantia nigra DA neurone degeneration).

Pathology of idiopathic PD Striatal loss of dopamine (putamen > caudate) (clinical presentation when DA loss >80%).

Melanin-containing cell bodies in pars compacta of substantia nigra undergo depigmentation (reduced pre-synaptic nigrostriatal DA production leads to diminished inhibition of striatal cholinergic neurones).

Depigmentation of locus coeruleus and vagus dorsal motor nucleus.

↓ cortical NA and that in locus coeruleus.

↓ CCK and substance P in substantia nigra.

↓ frontal cortex somatostatin.

Loss of neurones sometimes → diffuse cortical atrophy.

Reactive astrocytosis.

Lewy bodies (amorphous, electron-dense bodies with proteinaceous core):

– found in many structures but in particular; substantia nigra, locus coeruleus and dorsal motor nucleus of vagus.

Not characteristic of post-encephalitic PD or chemically induced parkinsonism.

(NB occasionally found in normal brain tissue and Alzheimer's disease.)

Clinically Classic triad of tremor, rigidity and bradykinesia.

'Simian' stoop and festinant (shuffling) gait. Reduced arm swing.

Expressionless, unblinking, mask-like face maintaining 'serpentine' stare.

Greasy skin (seborrhoea), excessive salivation and slurred, soft, sonorous voice.

Small handwriting (micrographia).

Psychological complications Depression (50%) – guilt is less common a feature and suicide rate is low.

Psychosis (10%) – delusions and visual hallucinations.

Dementia (15% of all patients, 40% of those >70 years old).

Cognitive deficits – bradyphrenia, visuospatial impairments, poor memory (especially recent) and abstract reasoning.

Huntington's disease (HD) (George Huntington, 1850–1916)

1 in 20 000 males and females equally affected. Typical onset 25 – 50 years of age.

Autosomal dominant genetic disorder. Excessive trinucleotide CAG repeats on short arm of chromosome 4 (normally about 9–39 repeats; HD associated with >40 repeats; the greater the number of repeats the younger the onset of disease).

Results in abnormal protein called huntingtin.

It is thought that the genetic defect affects NMDA receptor function and that this predisposes to Glutamate induced excitotoxicity.

Neuropathology:

Cerebral cortex atrophy especially frontal lobes.

Cortical neuronal loss affects layers III, V and VI.

Neuronal degeneration and loss associated with marked astrocytosis.

Ventricles are enlarged and are described as 'bat-wing ventricles'.

Marked caudate nucleus atrophy especially the head of the caudate. Begins medially and eventually interrupts cotico-striato-pallido-thalamic connections. Detectable by CT and MRI.

Degeneration of striatal GABA neurones ($\downarrow$ caudate (GABA) to <50% of normal) and reduction of glutamic acid decarboxylase activity (striatal $\downarrow$ of up to 85%).

PET shows early (prior to structural changes) caudate hypometabolism.

Loss of striatal enkephalinergic neurones (project to globus pallidus) and substance P containing neurones (project to substantia nigra).

Reduction in number of striatal aspartate receptors.

ACh levels ↓.

Somatostatin and neuropeptide Y levels ↑.

DA hypersensitivity.

Clinically HD produces changes of *m*ood, *m*otion and *m*entation.

Initial symptoms: 10% in childhood and 25% over the age of 50 years.

Emotional symptoms include anxiety, depression and irritability. Occasionally paranoid psychotic symptoms.

Motor symptoms include choreiform movements which are initially distal (piano-playing; milk-maids sign; jack in the box tongue), abnormal saccades, dystonia, tremor, dysarthria abnormality of gait (lurching and contorted).

Cognitive symptoms are those of insidious global dementia. Language function and memory are relatively spared.

Wilson's disease (hepatolenticular degeneration) (Wilson, S. 1878–1936) Autosomal recessive genetic disorder (chromosome 13).

Caeruloplasmin (copper carrying globulin) deficiency leads to copper deposition:

- cerebrum: dementia and emotional lability
- putamen: choreoathetosis, 'wing-beating' or 'bat-wing' tremor
- liver: cirrhosis, hepatosplenomegaly, jaundice
- eye:
    cornea (Descemet's membrane)
    lens (sunflower cataract)
    cornea (Kayser–Fleischer ring – outer margin of iris)

Clinically *ABCDE*

*A*thetosis
*B*ehavioural changes
*C*ognitive impairment
*D*ysphagia, *D*ysarthria and *D*rooling
*E*motional lability

Tics *PQRSt*

*P*urposeless, *Q*uick, *R*epetitive, *St*ereotyped movements of functionally related muscle groups

Described as simple (incomplete movements) or complex (complete movements) and can be motor or vocal. The frequency and intensity of tics is increased by anxiety, fatigue and excitement however, they can be consciously temporarily suppressed. Occur three times more often in boys. Peak age of onset 7 years. 90% remit spontaneously within 5 years.

Gilles de la Tourette's syndrome (Itard 1825)

STUV

*S*tereotypies (jumping, dancing)
*T*ics
*U*tterances (clicks, throat clearing, snorts, grunts)
*V*ocal tics (coprolalia, occasionally accompanied by copropraxia)

Associated with:

– obsessive–compulsive symptoms (50%)
– attention-deficit hyperactivity disorder (ADHD)
– soft neurological signs
– minor EEG abnormalities
– ↓ glucose metabolism (cingulate and inferior frontal cortex).

Neuroleptic-induced movement disorders

Acute onset Acute dystonia, oculogyric crisis, akathisia, Parkinsonism.

Tardive (late) onset Tardive dyskinesias, tics, oral-buccal-lingual syndrome, akathisia, dystonia, stereotypies.

Akathisia Regular, continuous leg movements (e.g. to and fro motion, crossing and uncrossing).

Tardive dyskinesia Irregular or stereotyped lower face, tongue and jaw movements. Associated with prolonged high-dose neuroleptic exposure and more common in women and with increasing age.

Neuropathology

Dementias

Alzheimer's disease (Alzheimer, A. 1864–1915)

Macroscopic changes

- shrunken gyri and widened sulci
- reduction of total brain weight (from in excess of 1200 g to less than 1000 g) because of symmetrical global cortical atrophy; greatest in medial temporal lobe especially parahippocampal gyrus (PHG)
- ventricular enlargement; greatest in temporal horns of lateral ventricles.

Microscopic changes

- loss of pyramidal neurones from cortical layers III and V (especially younger patients)
- reduction of neurophil and synaptic innervation ($\downarrow$ synaptophysin and synapsin 1)
- neurofibrillary tangles (see below)
- amyloid plaques (see below)
- astrocyte proliferation
- granulovacuolar degeneration, especially in hippocampal pyramidal cells
- Hirano bodies.

- **Amyloid (neuritic/senile) plaques** extracellular, insoluble core of beta-amyloid (A4 protein) fibrils (8 nm in diameter and 39–43 aa long) derived from amyloid precursor protein (APP), containing aluminium silicate and surrounded by degenerating neurites and astrocyte processes. Overall diameter up to 200 μm. Not specific to AD (also found in normal ageing, Down's syndrome, CJD and lead encephalopathy) but density correlates to severity of disease. APP gene is located on long arm of Chromosome 21.
- **Neurofibrillary tangles (NFTs)**: intraneuronal, necessary for histological diagnosis and numbers correlate to severity of illness. Less common in non-dements but can occur in normal ageing, Down's syndrome, progressive supranuclear palsy, postencephalitic Parkinson's disease, subacute sclerosing panencephalitis and dementia pugilistica.
  - NFTs contain both straight filaments and paired helical filaments (PHFs). Abnormal phosphorylation of microtubular-associated protein (MAP) tau, produces paired helical filament-tau (double-helix PHF-tau). Phosphorylated tau – 68 kD molecular weight

and also called A68 protein, Alzheimer's disease-associated protein (ADAP).
- Tau proteins associate with tubulin and alter cell shape. They are concentrated in neuronal axons.
• **Neurochemistry**: loss of basal forebrain (nucleus basalis of Meynert, medial septal nuclei and diagonal band of Broca) cholinergic cortical and hippocampal innervation.
- Reduction in choline acetyl-transferase (ChAT) and acetylcholinesterase (AChE).
- Pre-synaptic nicotinic receptor concentration is reduced. Muscarinic M1 receptor activity is normal.
- Reduced adrenergic and serotonergic cortical innervation:
    $\downarrow$ $5HT_2$ receptors in cortex (frontal, temporal, parietal) and hippocampus. Numbers of $5HT_2$ receptors and tangles inversely correlated and reduction of receptors is thought to be due to pyramidal cell loss.
    $\downarrow$ α_2 adrenoceptors in hippocampus (α_1 receptors unchanged and α adrenoceptors unaltered in frontal and temporal cortices)
    $\downarrow$ β_1 receptors and $\uparrow$ β_2 receptors in prefrontal cortex along with reduction of NA.
- Interneurone GABA levels are reduced (cortical loss of GABA re-uptake markers).
- Cortical and hippocampal Glutamate is reduced.
- Somatostatin (co-localizes with GABA) is reduced.
- Substance P, vasoactive intestinal peptide (VIP) and cholecystokinin (CCK) show no consistent changes.
- Activity of second messenger systems adenylate cyclase (G_s-linked) and phophoinositide is reduced in frontal cortex of AD patients.

Non-alzheimer dementias

Vascular dementia

Multi-infarct dementia

• Macroscopic changes:
  - localized/general brain atrophy
  - major vessel arteriosclerosis
  - ventricular enlargement
  - cerebral infarction* (cortical, subcortical, both) (infarction of specific brain regions, e.g. hippocampus or thalamus can in itself lead to dementia syndrome)
  - leukoaraiosis† (white matter rarefaction) (usually seen on CT scan or MRI).

* It is of note that there is usually no detectable cognitive impairment until 50 ml of brain tissue is affected and usually dementia ensues once the area affected exceeds 100 ml. Also left hemisphere lesions more likely to be associated with clinical dementia.

† Not specific for vascular dementias; found in 40% of normal elderly population.

● **Microscopic changes**:
  – cell changes of ischaemic infarction.

Binswanger disease (subacute arteriosclerotic encephalopathy) (Binswanger, O. 1852–1929)

● Macroscopic changes:
  – lacunes
  – subcortical white matter demyelination
  – major vessel arteriosclerosis
  – neuronal loss
  – etat crible
  – ventricular enlargement.
● **Microscopic changes**:
  – gliosis.

Congophilic (amyloid) angiopathy

● Macroscopic and microscopic changes:
  – Rare form of cerebral vessel specific amyloidosis with dominant inheritance. Associated with amyloid precursor protein gene mutation (Dutch family studies).
  – Amyloid deposits (AD) in cerebral blood vessels cause weakening and predispose to lobar intracerebral haemorrhages or can cause narrowing of vessels and stenosis leading to ischaemia.
  (NB Cerebral vessel amyloid deposition is seen in normal ageing and in up to 40% of AD.)

Lewy body dementia Lewy body: consists of dense core vesicles, MAP, tau protein, ubiquitin and protein neurofilaments.

Diffuse Lewy body disease

● Microscopic changes:
  – subcortical Lewy bodies
  – neuronal loss from subcortical nuclei – basal n. of Meynert, substantia nigra, locus coeruleus

- cortical Lewy bodies*
- senile plaques
- neurofibrillary tangles
- reduced cortical choline acetyl transferase (CAT)
* Temporal cortex, cingulate gyrus and parahippocampal gyrus particularly high content when compared to Lewy body concentrations in Parkinson's disease.

Frontal lobe dementias

Pick's disease (Pick, A. 1851–1924)

- Macroscopic changes:
  - mild generalized atrophy
  - marked asymmetrical fronto-temporal atrophy (sparing of posterior one-third superior temporal gyrus)
  - affects white and grey matter leading to characteristic brownish 'knife-blade' gyri with spongiform change (grey/white boundary is blurred and white matter has rubbery consistency)
  - occasional atrophy of caudate and putamen
  - ventricular enlargement.
- **Microscopic changes** (observed in cortex, basal ganglia, substantia nigra, locus coeruleus):
  - severe neuronal loss (particularly outer cortical layers)
  - proliferation of astrocytes
  - fibrous gliosis
  - Pick cells (swollen cortical pyramidal cells also called balloon cells)*
  - Pick's bodies (intraneuronal argyrophilic inclusions)*
  (* Present in up to one-third of cases. NB occasional distinction between Pick's disease (that with Pick cells and bodies) and frontal-lobe dementia (cases without these features). Distinction of limited use clinically.)
  (NB plaques, tangles and Lewy bodies absent.)

Subcortical and degenerative dementias

Progressive supranuclear palsy Slow dementing syndrome with prominent neurological signs of unknown aetiology occurring in late adult life.

- **Macroscopic and microscopic changes**:
  - neuronal loss
  - subcortical and brainstem tangles (consisting of straight filaments).

Huntington's disease

Wilson's disease

Hellervorden–Spatz disease (Martha–Alma disease) Rare recessive illness characterized by iron deposition in substantia nigra and globus pallidus.

- **Macroscopic changes**:
  - hypodensities seen on MRI scanning.
- **Microscopic changes**:
  - sea-blue histiocytes.

Prion diseases Altered prion proteins (PrP^c)

Creutzfeldt–Jakob disease

- Macroscopic changes:
  - brain atrophy is minimal if it occurs at all
  - can affect whole of CNS (especially spinal cord long descending tracts and anterior horn cells).
- **Microscopic changes**:
  - astrocyte proliferation
  - status spongiosus (cortical grey matter, basal ganglia, motor nuclei and thalamus)
  - neuronal degeneration and gliosis (without inflammation)
  - protease resistant prion protein (PrP^{sc}) accumulates in neurones and forms plaques.

Gerstmann–Straussler–Scheinker syndrome (spinocerebellar ataxia)

- Microscopic changes:
  - deposits akin to AD plaques containing scrapie amyloid protein.

Punch-drunk syndrome (boxing encephalopathy)

- Macroscopic changes:
  - ventricular enlargement
  - corpus callosum thinning
  - cerebral atrophy
  - septum pellucidum perforation.

- **Microscopic changes**:
  - neuronal degeneration
  - neurofibrillary tangles.

Cerebral tumours

1:20 000 in UK.

Second most common cause of cancer-related death in children less than 14 years of age.

- 80% primary cerebral tumours (make up 10% of all neoplasms);
  - 50% derived from neuroepithelial cells:
    gliomas (see below)
    primitive neuro-ectodermal tumours (medulloblastoma, neuroblastoma)
    lymphoid tumours
  - 25% mesodermal derivation
    menigiomas (often calcify)
    meningial sarcomas
  - remainder:
    ectodermal derivation (pituitary adenoma, craniopharyngioma)
    vascular tissue derivatives (haemangioblastomas)
    neurilemmomas (Schwannomas), Schwann cell derivatives.
  (70% of primary cerebral tumours: supratentorial in adults; *infra*-tentorial in *inf*ants and children (<14 yr of age)
- 20% secondary, metastases: primary tumour in – lung, breast, kidney, colon, ovary and prostate.

Gliomas: derived from glial cells

  - astrocytomas: commonest, grow diffusely, poorly encapsulated and graded I–IV. Grade IV (gliobastoma multiforme), most severe, has 3-year survival rate of 4%
  - oligodendrogliomas: slow growth, often calcify
  - ependymomas: slow growing in ventricular system and can be intracranial or spinal.

Effects of cerebral tumours:

  - local:
    focal signs: because of infiltration and destruction of tissue. May compromise circulation and cause oedema
    seizures: in about a third of cases, particularly if frontal or temporal lobes involved
  - generalized: raised intracranial pressure (ICP).

Raised intracranial pressure (ICP)

Mechanisms:

↑ brain volume
  - space occupying lesion
  - oedema: cytotoxic (toxins and hypoxia)
              vasogenic (excess extracellular fluid)
↑ cerebrospinal fluid (CSF)
  - obstruction of flow at any level
↑ intracranial blood volume
  - hypoxia
  - hypercapnia
  - trauma.

Signs and symptoms of ↑ ICP:

  - headache: worst in mornings; exacerbated by coughing, sneezing, stooping and caused by deformation of dura and blood vessels.
  - vomiting: upon waking
  - papilloedema: subarachnoid space extends along optic nerve
  - brain herniation: subfalcine; transtentorial; produce false localizing signs
  - rostrocaudal migration of brainstem: divided into stages. Diencephalic, mesencephalic, pontine and medullary reflects the progressive occlusion of brainstem blood vessels. At first the patient becomes drowsy slipping into an unconscious state and assuming a decerebrate posture. Blood pressure is raised and the heart rate falls (Cushing response). Pupils are initially dilated and fixed to light becoming **p**inpoint during the **p**ontine stage when the corneal reflexes are also lost. In the medullary stage the heart rate increases (tachycardia) and the blood pressure now falls. Respiration assumes a Cheyne–Stokes pattern and cardiac arrest is imminent.

(NB phenomenon of intracranial compliance – ICP increases can be buffered by displacement of CSF and blood.)

Epilepsy (see Figure 9.9)

Lifetime prevalence 2%.

Two-thirds partial (commonest temporal lobe epilepsy – TLE) remainder generalized and mixed.

Causes ICTAL

75% *I*diopathic
9% *C*erebrovascular accident (CVA)

7% *t*rauma
6% *A*lcohol

Other causes: drugs, infections, malformations, degenerative and metabolic diseases.

Epileptic personality *PERSON*

*P*edantic
*E*gocentric
*R*eligiose
*S*low in thought ('viscous')
*O*bsessional
'k*N*it-picking' – critical

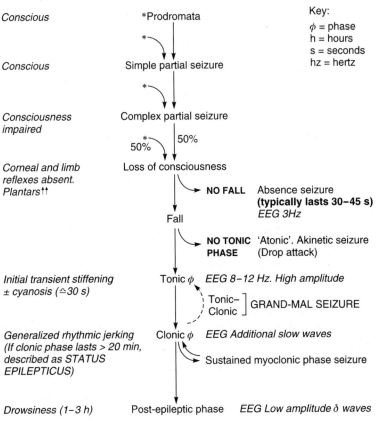

* Starting points

Key:
ϕ = phase
h = hours
s = seconds
hz = hertz

Figure 9.9 *Epilepsy*

Psychiatric aspects of epilepsy

- Ictal prodrome

  STIRS

  ↓ *S*leep
  ↑ *T*ension
  ↑ *I*rritability
  ↑ *R*estlessness
  *S*uicidal ideation and depression

- Ictal: automatisms, fugues, twilight states.
- Inter-ictal:
  - aggressive behaviour – *E*pisodic *D*yscontrol *S*yndrome

    *E*EG changes, *D*isorder of personality, *S*enseless aggression and violence

  - depression and risk of suicide ↑x4
  - schizophreniform psychosis (controversial associations)
    *n*ormal pre-morbid personality preserved
    *n*ice: warmer affect than in schizophrenia
    *n*egative family history of schizophrenia
    *n*eurological abnormalities ↑
    *n*ot distinguishable from schizophrenia on basis of psychopathology.

Schizophrenia

Macroscopic and microscopic neuropathology from post-mortem and histological studies and structural and functional neuroimaging:

↓ brain mass and length
↓ cerebral grey matter volume (5–10% reduction); especially temporal lobe; superior temporal gyrus is smaller particularly on left side
↓ size of cingulate and parahippocampal gyri
↓ size of hippocampus and amygdala (>on left)
↑ size of septum pellucidum with greater incidence of cavum septum pellucidum
↓ hippocampal neuronal size and mossy cell fibre staining displacement of pre-alpha and pre-beta-cells in entorhinal cortex
↓ neuronal density in anterior cingulate, primary motor and prefrontal cortices and thalamic medial dorsal nucleus, the cerebellum and nucleus accumbens
no significant gliosis.

Depression

Neurotransmitter and receptor changes:

- ↓ noradrenergic function in depressives
- ↓ growth hormone response to clonidine (post-synaptic NA receptor down-regulation)
- ↓ CSF MHPG
- ↓ platelet cAMP turnover (with clonidine stimulation).

Serotonergic function in depressives:

- ↓ plasma tryptophan (NB tryptophan depletion of recovered depressives continuing treatment causes temporary relapse)
- ↓ platelet 5-HT uptake presynaptically
- ↑ platelet imipramine binding 5-HT$_2$ post-synaptically
- ↓ CSF 5-HIAA (more so in those with a history of suicide and particularly those using violent methods) (NB thought to be associated with impulsive behaviour and also found in schizophrenia and personality disorders).
- ↓ cortisol response to ipsapirone challenge

Neuropathology of chronic alcohol abuse

Seizures (10% of alcoholics) due to:

- – direct toxicity of alcohol
- – head injury
- – withdrawal
- – hypoglycaemia.

Peripheral neuropathy (10%) because of thiamine (B1) deficiency.

Cerebellar degeneration Affects vermis and causes gait disturbance.

Wernicke–Korsakoff syndrome Acute and chronic degenerative changes; caused by petechial haemorrhage, parenchymal degeneration and capillary proliferation of gray matter surrounding II and IV ventricles.

(Mamillary bodies, hypothalamus, thalamus (dorso-medial nucleus), periaqueductal grey).

Optic atrophy Because of vitamin B deficiency, associated heavy smoking, consumption of methanol.

Central pontine myelinolysis Progressive demyelination of pontine (central) structures. Pseudobulbar palsy and spasticity.

Marchiafava–Bignami disease (Especially red wine) demyelination of corpus callosum, cerebellar peduncles, optic tracts and cerebral hemisphere white matter. Leads to cognitive impairment, dementia, emotional lability, fits.

Myopathy (Particularly proximal.)

10 Neurophysiology

Sleep

Recurrent, regular, reversible state characterized by quiescence and diminished responsiveness to external stimuli.

The EEG in an awake individual is random and fast. When resting quietly, with eyes closed, the EEG shows alpha waves. Muscle tone, measured by electromyogram (EMG) activity, is high and eye movements are present. The transition through drowsiness from being awake to sleeping is called the **hypnagogic period** and during this muscle tone diminishes, the eyes begin to roll and EEG alpha activity decreases.

Sleep is divided into **REM (rapid eye movement)** and non-REM sleep. REM sleep is also called desynchronized sleep and dreaming sleep.

The normal pattern of sleep involves 4–5 cycles of alternating REM and non-REM sleep with REM sleep becoming progressively more prominent. The total time spent in REM sleep is 90 minutes in adults (20% of total sleep period).

Other than brief periods of wakefulness (5% of total sleep period) the remaining time is spent in non-REM sleep (75%).

Non-REM sleep

Consists of four stages (after Rechtschaffen akales):

- **Stage 1** (5%): As the individual falls asleep alpha activity diminishes to less than 50% of the EEG record giving way to characteristic low-amplitude, low-voltage **theta** activity. Occasional vertex sharp waves (V waves) are normal. EMG activity decreases and rolling eye movements are present.
- **Stage 2** (55%): Now in light sleep the EEG shows low voltage, slow frequencies (theta waves) that are interrupted intermittently by **K complexes** and **sleep spindles**. The latter are spindle-shaped EEG traces of short bursts (0.5 s) of waves (12–14 Hz). K complexes are high-voltage spikes consisting of a negative wave followed 0.75 s later by a positive wave.
- **Stage 3** (5%): The onset of deep sleep is accompanied by the appearance on EEG of high amplitude (75 µV), low frequency (2 Hz) **delta waves**, which by definition form less than 50% but more than 20% of the trace.
- **Stage 4** (10%): Delta waves form more than **50%** of EEG activity.

Collectively stages 3 and 4 are called **slow wave sleep** or **synchronized sleep**. Sleep spindles can occur in slow wave sleep.

REM sleep

The EEG in REM sleep is characterized by random, fast mixed frequency activity of low-voltage (similar to awake state) hence it is also called **paradoxical sleep**. It is distinguished by **saw-tooth waves**.

Sleep can be plotted as a **hypnogram**. In a normal adult the pattern of sleep is as follows:

After entering sleep the individual progresses through stages 1–4 and then returns to stages 3 and then 2. From stage 2 having been asleep for about 90 minutes the individual enters their first period of REM sleep. The individual then reverts to stage 2 sleep and the cycle is repeated 4–5 times during the night with each cycle lasting 90 minutes. As sleep progresses the proportion of REM sleep increases and that of slow-wave sleep decreases.

Sleep changes with age

Newborn sleeps 16 hours a day and is able to pass directly from wakefulness into REM sleep, which takes up more than 50% of sleep. By 4 months REM forms 40% of total sleep and is usually preceded by non-REM sleep.

A young adult sleeps 8 hours a day of which 90 minutes (approx. 20%) is REM sleep.

Table 10.1 Differences between REM and non-REM sleep

	REM	Non-REM
Autonomic activity	Sympathetic	Parasympathetic
Heart rate	↑	↓
Blood pressure	↑	↓
Cerebral blood flow	↑	↓
Respiratory rate	↑	↓
Dreaming	↑	↓
Erection (penis)	Yes	–
Myoclonic jerks	Yes	–
Muscular tone	↓↓	↓
Ocular movements	Yes	Few

Neurochemical correlates of sleep

Sleep is promoted by – ACH(REM), GABA.

Sleep is inhibited by – NA, SHT, DOP, Histamine.

Neuroendocrine correlates of sleep*

as sleep sTarTs – Testosterone levels ↑
Prolactin Peaks Prior to waking (↑ last two hours of sleep)
REM sleep – ↓ REnin and ↓ Melatonin
Slow-wave Sleep – peaks of SomatoStatin (SS)

Growth Hormone levels – High Cortisal levels – Low

Sleep–wake cycle

Two main theories:

1 Cellular (Hobson's) model Involves three groups of central neurones:

Nucleus reticularis pontis caudalis (gigantocellular tegmental field of pons) cholinergic neurones function as 'on' cells promoting REM sleep.

Dorsal raphe nuclei serotonergic neurones and locus coeruleus noradrenergic neurones function as 'off' cells and a gradual increase in their activity inhibits the REM promoting cholinergic cells and allows slow-wave sleep to resume.

There is little support for this model.

2 Monoaminergic (Jouvet's, two-stage or biochemical) model Slow-wave sleep (non-REM) is associated with Raphe complex Serotonergic neuronal activity. Destruction of these neurones leads to insomnia. Serotonin precursor tryptophan is hypnotic.

Locus coeruleus noradrenergic neuronal activity associated with REM sleep. Destruction leads to selective REM suppression.

Lesion effects Elimination of all somatosensory inputs by sectioning below medulla (encephale isole) preserves normal sleep-wake cycle.

Mid-pontine transection leads to being permanently awake.

Mid-collicular brainstem transection leads to permanent sleep.

Hence arousal area above sleep promoting area.

EEG

In 1929 Hans Berger first described electroencephalography as a safe means of investigating brain function. The standard electroencephalogram (EEG) involves recording from electrodes placed on the scalp according to the international 10–20 system.

Normally 40 electrodes are applied using the nasion, inion and left and right auricular depressions as landmarks and recording is done from 8 or 16 channels.

A standard EEG recording includes:

- several minutes at rest (and perhaps sleep)
- whilst overbreathing (hyperventilation)
- during exposure to flashing lights (photic stimulation).

Activating procedures provoke abnormalities.

The normal activity range is 1–40 Hz frequency and 5–150 microvolts amplitude.

EEG is useful in diagnosing, defining and monitoring the treatment of epilepsy.

However, a *no*rmal EEG does *no*t exclude epilepsy.

Specialized forms of recording allow measurement of activity from specific parts of the brain e.g. nasopharyngeal and sphenoidal recordings detect medial temporal lobe activity.

Type of recording	Electrode placement
Sphenoidal	– between zygoma and mandibular coronoid notch
Nasopharyngeal	– superior nasopharynx
Electrocorticography	– surface of the brain
Depth electroencephalography	– inside the brain

Other means of recording the EEG:

- ambulatory EEG – record is maintained on suitable portable recorder
- video and event recorders can be used to correlate clinical findings with those of EEG
- telemetric recording provides a record from a distance.

Normal EEG wave patterns: (classified according to frequency Hz)

BATHED

Beta:	>13
Alpha:	8–13
***THE*ta:**	4–8
Delta:	<4

- Beta activity (β): awake resting adult with open eyes. Activity is related to sensory-motor cortical stimulation and is enhanced by anxiety. Best recorded from frontocentral positions. Variance according to cortical site described as **desynchronization** (simultaneous waves are out of phase). Beta displacement of alpha activity upon arousal is called **alerting** or **arousal response** and described as **alpha blocking**.

- Alpha activity (α): awake resting adult EEG pattern that is most prominent over the occipital region. It is accentuated by eye closure and attenuated by attention. It has a circadian rhythm and varies according to menstrual cycle. Amplitude can be attenuated by a fall in temperature and augmented by an increase. Its frequency diminishes with age and an inter-hemispheric difference of 1 Hz is pathological.

- Theta activity (θ): unusual in waking adult (found transiently in 15% of individuals). Normal in children aged 2–5 years and can be evoked by frustration. Also found in psychopaths.

- Delta activity (δ): abnormal in waking adult may signify brain neoplasm. Characteristic of deep sleep and common in children particularly infants. Induced by overbreathing. Diffuse cortical distribution.

- *L*ambda activity (λ): single, occipital sharp waves associated with ocular movements during visual scanning (associated with *l*ooking).

- *M*u activity (μ): arch-like waves that occur over precentral (*m*otor) cortex. Related to *m*ovement and mitigated by motion of contralateral limb.

- V waves: normal phenomenon of sharp electronegative waves that occur over the vertex in response to an auditory stimulus. Also seen in drowsiness.

- Spikes: brief peaks of less than 80 ms duration.

- Sharp waves: prominent wave formations of 80–200 ms duration.

EEG variance with age:

- full-term *n*ew-born EEG activity is almost *n*il
- infant (<1 yr) EEG desynchronized delta activity
- *t*oddler (>2 yr) EEG *t*heta activity predominates
- *a*dolescent (second decade of life) EEG *a*lpha activity is established
- *a*geing adult *a*lpha activity *a*ttenuates in *a*mplitude and frequency
- focal anterior temporal delta activity occurs in third of those over 60 yr.

Activating procedures: used to elicit EEG abnormalities not discernible in standard EEG:

- hyperventilation: cerebral hypoxia ⇒ cortical hyperexcitability

- photic stimulation (photic driving): (20–30 Hz) synchronizes alpha rhythm
- sleep deprivation.

EEG changes

May signify pathology and can sometimes be diagnostic (see below).

Can be because of surgical interventions, ECT and medication.

About 15% of EEG abnormalities are false positives.

EEG artefacts can be caused by:

- muscular contraction (local)
- eye movement
- cardiac arrhythmias.

Pathology

Organic psychoses (haemorrhage, infarction, infection, trauma, metabolic or endocrine disorders)

- usually diffuse symmetrical changes: $\downarrow \alpha$ and $\uparrow \delta$ and θ
- focal lesions, e.g. tumours, subdural haematoma EEG changes asymmetrical
- (NB non-organic stupor, e.g. because of depression or schizophrenia alpha activity is preserved).

Epilepsy Temporal lobe (TLE) sleep EEG + routine EEG detect spike foci in 90%.

Petit mal – generalized compound waves and spikes with frequency of 3Hz.

Dementias Alzheimer's – 95% of those with definite AD have abnormal EEG. Alpha activity decreases and delta/theta activity increases.

Multi-infarct dementia – EEG of little help.

Pick's disease – 50% have abnormal EEG. Alpha activity better preserved than in AD.

Infections HIV – diffuse slowing.

Subacute sclerosing panencephalitis (SSP) – bilateral, symmetrical and synchronous high amplitude polyphasic sharp wave and slow wave complexes in burst of up to **10 seconds** often accompanied by myoclonic jerks.

Herpes simplex encephalitis – **1–3 second** repetitive episodic discharges along with temporal lobe focal slow waves.

Creutzfeld–Jakob disease Bilateral, synchronous generalized irregular spike-wave complexes occurring at intervals of **0.5–1.0** seconds, often accompanied by myoclonic jerks. EEG is always abnormal. (cf. Description of SSP.)

Huntingdon's chorea Characteristic (not specific) diffuse flattening of EEG with low amplitude theta and delta waves.

Hepatic encephalopathy Triphasic waves and widespread slowing.

Hypoxia Occipital alpha rhythm is gradually replaced by theta and delta activity. Then with severe hypoxia there is initially intermittent cortical suppression resulting in a 'burst-suppression' effect which then progressively gives way to a flat EEG trace.

Midbrain tegmentum infarction Severe brainstem injury results in invariant alpha rhythm (alpha-coma).

Medication and physical treatments

Change	Medications		
↑β	Barbiturates	Benzodiazepines	TCAs
↑θ	Barbiturates	Benzodiazepines	TCAs Neuroleptics
↑δ			TCAs Neuroleptics

Alcohol increases alpha activity. Delirium tremens – increased fast activity.

Carbamazepine increases slow-wave sleep.

Lithium may produce focal slow waves in proportion to concentration.

ECT – between treatments there is diffuse EEG slowing (frontal region slowest to recover) increasing with each treatment and normalizing one month post-ECT.

Psychosurgery – increased bi-frontal delta activity.

Evoked potentials

Repeated stimulation of sensory modality results in neuronal, brainstem and cortical electrical responses which can only be discerned from background activity by signal averaging. Electrical responses are measured as evoked potentials (EP) typically consisting of a negative and positive component (negative upgoing and positive downgoing). Components are labelled according to their latency (time form stimulus to peak deflection) and direction of deflection:

e.g. P100 – positive peak 100 ms after stimulus.

Types of evoked potentials

VEPs (visual EP) – e.g. increase in latency of P100 on exposure to patterned stimulus (chess board) in individual with optic neuritis because of multiple sclerosis.

AEPs (auditory EP).

SEPs (somatosensory EP).

Following a stimulus:

- Short potential (<20 ms): corresponds to sensory pathway activity.
- Late potential (70–200 ms): cortical arrival and elaboration of sensory information.
- Cognitive potential (>200 ms): more complex processing of information, e.g. **P300** an event-related potential (ERP), seen 300–500 ms following stimulation and possibly relates to cognition and the formation of memory. P300 is maximal over parietal cortex regardless of sensory modality. It is altered in Down's syndrome, of diminished amplitude in autism, schizophrenia and Alzheimer's disease and larger in developmental dysphasia. The changes are not specific.
- **Contingent negative variation (CNV):** like P300, is an event-related slow potential that is elicited by initially providing a priming stimulus and then one which requires a response. It is also called the **expectancy wave** and consists of a slow negative potential shift particularly in frontal areas and vertex. Correlates to attention and motivation and is therefore attenuated by lack of stimulation and drugs such as barbiturates.
- **Bereitschaftspotential (readiness potential):** slow negative potential precedes voluntary movement by 1 second.

Novel techniques

Brain electrical activity mapping (BEAM)

EEG or EP data presented as maps, allowing summation, averaging and statistical analysis of such information.

Magnetoencephalography (MEG)

Involves the measurement of magnetic fields created by brain electrical potentials. It is a type of functional imaging with very low latency.

Action potential (AP) (see Figure 10.1)

The neuronal cell membrane has differential permeabilities that help create a negative **resting membrane potential** of -70 mV. This is essential for neuronal function (**excitability**). The resting membrane potential is closer to the **equilibrium potential** (balance of electrical

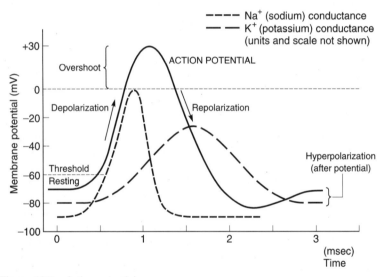

Figure 10.1 *Action potential*

potential and concentration gradient) of K^+ (-90 mV) than Na^+ as the resting membrane is more permeable to K^+. The **Na^+–K^+ ATPase pump** actively transports cations across the neuronal membrane ($3Na^+$ out for every $2K^+$ in) making a small direct contribution to the membrane potential because of this outward transfer of cations and a more significant indirect contribution by maintaining the ion concentration gradients.

Action potentials (AP) are rapid changes in the membrane potential involving transient (approx. 1 ms) local depolarization and repolarization. An AP can be:

- spontaneous (pacemaker activity)
- in response to activation of receptors
- because of synaptic stimulation.

NB transmission along axons is electrical, that across synapses is chemical.

The AP begins with rapid depolarization. During this 0.2–0.5 ms phase the permeability to Na^+ increases by a factor of 600 (activation) with initially insignificant change in K^+ permeability which lags behind. Na^+ ions therefore enter the neurone causing further depolarization and the membrane potential tends towards the equilibrium potential of Na^+ (+60 mV). Transiently the membrane polarity is reversed resulting in an 'overshoot'. Na^+ permeability is then inactivated and simultaneously K^+ permeability increases. Na^+ inactivation and the efflux of K^+ returns the membrane potential towards its resting value.

(NB the actual numbers of ions involved is extremely small and there is no change in the concentration gradients across the neuronal membrane during an AP.)

A typical AP lasts 1 ms. It is divided into several components.

To elicit an AP the membrane must depolarize beyond a critical level (threshold potential). For a typical neurone the threshold potential may be –60 mV and a stimulus that fails to depolarize the membrane to this level cannot elicit an AP. (NB axon hillock has lowest critical threshold.) However, an adequate stimulus can also fail to elicit an AP if the membrane is in its refractory period having been recently stimulated. The refractory period consists of an **absolute refractory period** (1 ms) **(ARP)** during which regardless of stimulus strength an AP cannot be elicited and a **relative refractory period** (10 ms) **(RRP)** in which a very large stimulus may be able to elicit an AP. The ARP corresponds to Na^+ inactivation. The RRP corresponds to after hyperpolarization.

The propagation of an AP involves repeated axonal depolarization. Its velocity is dependent upon axonal diameter and myelination.

As diameter ↑s so velocity ↑s. Myelination insulates membrane changes and causes APs to occur only at points of unmyelinated axon (**nodes of Ranvier**) resulting in **saltatory conduction**. Conduction velocities range from 1–100 ms^{-1}.

Nerve fibres are classified by a variety of conventions (Tables 10.2, 10.3):

Table 10.2 Classification of nerve fibres

Nerve fibres	Diameter (μm)	Conduction velocity ms⁻¹	Function
A (α)	12–20	70–120	Motor somatic; proprioception
A (β)	5–12	30–70	Touch; pressure; kinaesthesia
A (γ)	3–7	15–30	Touch; pressure; motor
A (δ)	1–5	12–30	Pain; pressure; temperature
B	1–3	3–15	Preganglionic (autonomic)
C	up to 1	<2	Pain
C	up to 1	<2	Postganglionic (sympathetic)

Table 10.3 Alternative classification of nerve fibres

Nerve fibres	Diameter (μm)	Conduction velocity ms⁻¹	Function
Ia	12	70–120	Muscle spindle afferents
Ib			Tendon organs
II	10	25–70	Skin mechanoreceptors
III	3	10–25	Muscle deep pressure sensors
IV	1	1	Pain fibres (unmyelinated)

Synapse (see Figure 10.2)

Specialized junction between two neurone (NB synapse with muscle–neuromuscular junction or plate).

Usually involves:

axon	and	dendrites	(axodendritic) but can involve
axon		cell body	(axonsomatic)
axon		axon	(axoaxonal)
dendrite		dendrite	(dendrodentritic)

The neurones involved are called **pre-synaptic** or **post-synaptic** depending on whether they carry APs towards or away from the synapse. Functionally synapses are of two types. Most synapses are chemical and rely on pre-synaptic release of neurotransmitters. Electrical synapses have direct membranous contact at **gap junctions** and transmit information faster than chemical synapses. **Conjoint synapses** have both chemical and electrical characteristics.

Chemical synapse neurotransmission:

The pre-synaptic neurone ends as a swelling called the **synaptic (terminal) bouton** or synaptic knob. This contains membrane-enclosed vesicles which store a chemical neurotransmitter. The pre-synaptic neurone is separated from the post-synaptic neurone by a **synaptic cleft** (200 Angstroms). The arrival of a pre-synaptic AP causes Ca^{2+} influx which

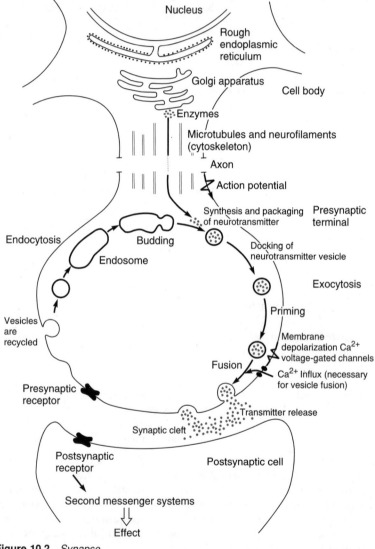

Figure 10.2 *Synapse*

initiates and assists pre-synaptic vesicle migration and fusion leading to synaptic cleft neurotransmitter release. The neurotransmitter diffuses across the synaptic cleft to combine with post-synaptic receptors. Neurotransmitter binding results in post-synaptic membrane permeability changes. The whole process takes 1 ms to occur and this is called the synaptic delay. Neurotransmitter inactivation terminates synaptic activity.

Synapses can be excitatory or inhibitory depending upon the characteristics of the neurotransmitter. An excitatory post-synaptic potential (EPSP) causes depolarization while an inhibitory post-synaptic potential (IPSP) causes hyperpolarization. EPSPs and IPSPs are electrotonic potentials (amplitude diminishes with increasing distance from site of initiation) and can be summated. This integration is necessary as a single EPSP (of 1 mV) is insufficient to reach an AP threshold. Potentials can combine temporally (temporal summation) and spatially (spatial summation). However, repeated stimulation at some synapses can result in diminishing post-synaptic potentials.

This is called **post-tetanic depression**. Partial restriction of calcium influx augments the potentials, called **post-tetanic facilitation**, following which there is a brief increase in the size of the response called **post-tetanic potentiation**. Hippocampal post-tetanic potentiation can last several hours and is called **long-term potentiation (LTP)**. LTP involves L-glutamate and is associated with memory.

Synapses are unidirectional and ensure that APs (which propagate in both directions along the membrane) result in one-way neurotransmission along nerve fibres.

Peripheral receptors

Receptors sense the external and internal environments. The sensory elements presented to receptors determine their characteristics and they are named accordingly.

Almost all receptors can be activated by more than one form of stimulus. However, they are specifically more sensitive to one kind of stimulus.

- Exteroceptors: e.g. receptors in skin sense immediate environment
- Telereceptors: e.g. eyes and ears sense distant environment
- Nociceptors: receptive to pain
- Thermoreceptors: receptive to temperature
- Mechanoreceptors: sense vibration and touch
- Proprioceptors: sense position.

Receptors can be specialized nerve endings or distinct cellular structures connected to nerves.

Skin receptors

- Pacinian corpuscle: pressure
- Free nerve ending: pressure, touch, pain, temperature
- Merkel's disks: pressure, touch
- Peritrichial arborization: pressure, touch
- Meissner's corpuscle: touch, discrimination
- Ruffini ending: pressure, touch, temperature
- Krause's corpuscles: temperature.

In mechanoreceptors such as the Pacinian corpuscle receptor activation results in an initial depolarization called the **generator potential** (GP). This is very different to an AP.

Table 10.4 Action and generator potentials

	Action potential	*Generator potential*
Duration (ms)	1–2	1–2
Refractory period	Yes (ARP 1 ms)	No
Conduction	Active; no loss of amplitude	Passive; amplitude decreases
Summation	No	Yes
Response	All-or-none	Graded

GP amplitude determines AP frequency only.

GP amplitude varies according to:

- intensity of stimulus
- its rate of change in application
- adaptation
- summation.

Thus sensory transduction is amplitude-dependent whereas transmission of information is frequency-coded. Subsequent processing of sensory information includes **lateral inhibition,** which allows the introduction of contrast by restricting the lateral spread of a stimulus amongst parallel inputs.

Adaptation is the reduction in AP frequency despite continuing stimulation. It occurs in both phasic and tonic receptors.

An increase in intensity of a stimulus can be coded by increased AP frequency and by activation of additional receptors/neurones. This is called **recruitment**.

Motor reflexes

Motor unit

Comprises a motor neurone axon and the muscle fibres it supplies. The innervation ratio (muscle fibres: innervating axons) which varies (4 in eye muscles up to 2000 in postural muscles) determines the degree of muscular control. The force of contraction of a muscle is increased by increasing recruitment of motor units and then their discharge frequency.

Stretch reflex (myostatic)

Stretch receptors called muscle spindles lie parallel to muscle fibres and are activated by lengthening of muscles. Annulospiral (primary) endings connect directly via Ia afferents to motor neurones and when stimulated cause contraction of the muscle. Important in tone/posture and movement.

Intrafusal muscle spindle → 1a neurones → spinal cord → extrafusal and motor neurone.

Clasp-knife reflex (inhibitory)

Golgi tendon organs respond to muscle contraction and inhibit via Ib afferents to motor neurones further muscle contraction. Important in protecting and controlling muscular tension.

Golgi tendon organs → 1b neurones → spinal cord → α motor neurone inhibition.

11 *Neurochemistry*

Neurotransmitters

Neurotransmitters are released at neuronal synapses whereupon they bind to specific receptors to produce specific responses. To be defined as a neurotransmitter it must be present in neuronal endings along with the necessary means for its synthesis and degradation.

Neurotransmitters are stored in pre-synaptic vesicles and released into the synaptic cleft in response to a stimulus. This is a Ca^{2+}-dependent process involving the fusion of neurotransmitter vesicles with specific pre-synaptic areas.

Of the neurotransmitters important to psychiatry, acetylcholine (ACh), serotonin (5-hydroxytryptamine, 5-HT) and the catecholamines nora-drenaline (NA) and dopamine (DA) will be discussed in detail by illustrating their synthesis, degradation and actions. The amino-acids gamma-aminobutyric acid (GABA) and glutamate also have important neurotransmitter functions, as do some peptides (vasoactive intestinal peptide, endorphins, cholecystokinin, somatostatin, neurotensin).

Acetylcholine (see Figure 11.1)

Synthesis Acetylcholine (ACh) is synthesized in a single reaction:

choline + acetyl CoA ⇔ acetylcholine + coenzyme A

This is catalysed by **choline acetyltransferase (ChAT)** which is selective for cholinergic neurones in the nervous system. ChAT is synthesized in the rough endoplasmic reticulum of the perikaryon and taken via axoplasmic transport to the axon terminals where it is mostly free in the cytoplasm.

The rate of ACh synthesis is dependent upon the catalytic activity of ChAT, which in turn is primarily dependent upon the availability of choline. This ChAT is not in itself rate limiting. ChAT activity is altered by neuronal activity and is inhibited by ACh (product inhibition) through an allosteric ACh binding site on the enzyme. When ACh binds to ChAT it alters the three-dimensional conformation of the molecule and reduces its catalytic activity.

Choline is found in food such as vegetables, seeds, egg yolk and liver. It is also produced in the liver and transported across the blood–brain barrier (BBB) by a specific bi-directional carrier system situated in the endothelial cells of the capillaries. A low-affinity choline uptake

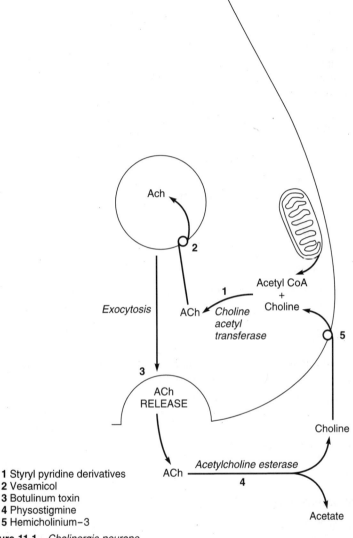

Figure 11.1   *Cholinergic neurone*

mechanism exists in all cells and the choline is used for the synthesis of phospholipids.

In the brain choline is used for the synthesis of phosphatidylcholine and ACh. A large proportion of choline is recycled as it is retrieved following the degradation of ACh by a sodium dependent, high-affinity, carrier-mediated mechanism that is specific to cholinergic neurones.

Coenzyme A contains adenine, a purine nucleotide base, and is found in mitochondria. Addition of an acetyl group to its sulphydryl group produces acetyl CoA.

Acetyl CoA is synthesized by the mitochondrial pyruvate dehydrogenase complex using pyruvate derived from glycolysis. Acetyl CoA is mainly used in the TCA cycle for the generation of energy, in the form of ATP. However, some is used for cytoplasmic ACh synthesis.

ACh storage/release ACh is stored in vesicles that originate in the cell body. These are transported to the nerve terminals and after ACh release they are recycled. There are two populations of ACh vesicles:

- VP_1 – reserve vesicles that are large and of low density
- VP_2 – recycled vesicles that are small and dense.

ACh inactivation Two means:

- diffusion out of synaptic cleft
- degradation.

   ACh + H_2O →* choline + acetic acid (*cholinesterase)

Cholinesterases Acetylcholinesterase (AChE) and butyrylcholinesterase (BChE).

Both are found in both brain and muscle. BChE (pseudocholinesterase) is found in brain glial cells, blood and liver.

AChE has greater specificity for ACh and is found in cholinergic neurones. It is a glycoprotein with two binding sites (anionic and esteratic). ACh degradation is a two-stage process involving a transient unstable intermediate acetylated AChE in which the enzyme is covalently bound via serine.

The action of drugs

- ACh synthesis:
  - **hemicholinium-3** and **triethylcholine:** inhibit high-affinity choline uptake. Choline lecithin are acetyl precusors which increase turnover.
- ACh storage/release:
  - **vesamicol:** inhibits vesicular transport
  - **α-latrotoxin:** (venom of black widow spider) depletes vesicles
  - **clostridial neurotoxins:** botulinum/tetanus disrupt vesicle exocytosis.
  - 3,4 diaminpyridine and phosphatidylserine promote ACh release.

- ACh mimetics:
  - carbachol, pilocarpine and bethanechol act on post-synaptic receptors (see Receptors).
- ACh degradation:
  - reversible/competitive anticholinesterases
    edrophonium: used diagnostically (myasthenia gravis)
    physostigmine: treatment of glaucoma
    neostigmine: does not cross BBB
  - long acting **tacrine** and clonepazil treatment of Alzheimer's disease
  - irreversible anticholinesterases:
    malathion, parathion
    nerve gases (sarin, tabun and di-isopropyl fluorophosphate).

Catecholamines (dopamine, noradrenaline and adrenaline)

Catecholamines are monoamines (dopamine, DA; noradrenaline, NA; and adrenaline, Ad) that possess the catechol group. DA, NA and adrenaline (Ad) share a common synthetic pathway illustrated in Figures 11.2 and 11.3.

The rate-limiting enzyme in the synthetic pathway is **tyrosine hydroxylase** (TH). TH consists of four identical subunits and contains Fe^{2+} ions that are essential for its activity. Also necessary is the pteridine cofactor, tetrahydrobiopterin (THB_4). Catecholamine synthesis can be inhibited by inhibitors of TH. This can be achieved by:

- chelation of Fe^{2+} ions
- competitive inhibition at pteridine binding site
- competitive inhibition at tyrosine binding site.

α-**methyl-para-tyrosine (AMPT)** binds at tyrosine binding site to inhibit TH.

Note that progression from dopamine to NA and Ad is dependent upon having the necessary enzymes.

Both acute and long-term mechanisms are used to regulate TH.

Acute mechanisms:

- end-product inhibition (catecholamines inhibit TH)
- stimulation-induced activation: neural activity increases enzyme hydroxylation by increasing the maximum velocity of the reaction and decreasing the effect of end-product inhibition
- enzyme activation by phosphorylation of regulatory serine residues:
  ser-19 – Ca^{2+} and calmodulin-dependent protein kinase II (CaM-K II)
  ser-31 – extracellular signal-regulated kinases (ERKs)
  ser-40 – cAMP-dependent protein kinase
- substrate availability – only of importance at high rates of activity.

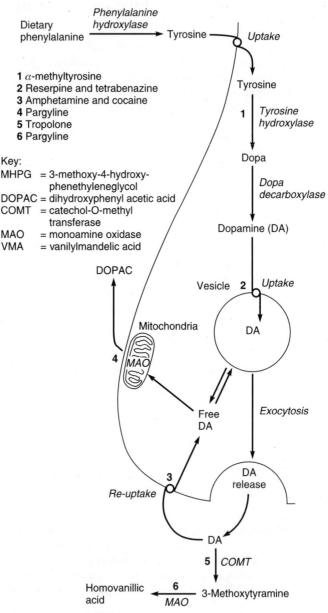

Figure 11.2 *Dopaminergic neurone*

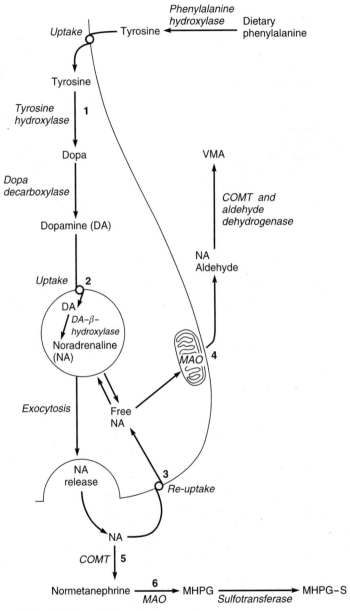

Figure 11.3 *Noradrenergic neurone*

Long-term mechanism:

- trans-synaptic induction: following stressful stimuli (e.g. cold, reserpine depletion) TH gene transcription and synthesis is increased.

Catecholamine storage Prior to synaptic release catecholamines are stored in vesicles. In addition to the catecholamine other vesicular constituents are ascorbic acid, calcium, nucleotides, chromogranins and dopamine β-hydroxylase (DBH). The necessary proteins are synthesized in the smooth endoplasmic reticulum (smER) and transferred to the Golgi apparatus where they undergo post-translational modification (addition of sulphate, phosphate or carbohydrate groups). The vesicles form by budding from the Golgi apparatus. ATP is transported into the vesicles and cytoplasmic dopamine is actively taken up. Within the vesicle DA can then be converted to NA which can subsequently be converted to Ad in the cytoplasm. For this latter step, NA moves into the cytoplasm and, once converted, Ad is taken up by the vesicle.

The uptake of catecholamines into secretory vesicles is dependent upon a vesicular membrane proton-translocating ATPase which moves protons into the vesicle. This creates an intra-vesicular pH of ~5.5 and an electrical potential such that there is a combined electrochemical gradient favouring the movement of catecholamines into the vesicles.

The catecholamine transporters can be inhibited by **tetrabenazine** and **reserpine**.

Catecholamine release Catecholamine release follows Ca^{2+}-dependent exocytosis and occurs in response to stimulation (membrane depolarization) and can therefore be inhibited by **tetrodotoxin** (**TTX**) (blocks Na^+ channels). Catecholamine release is stimulated by **methylphenidate** and **amphetamine.**

Catecholamine inactivation Catecholamine effects are terminated by uptake and catabolism.

Synaptic uptake: Na^+/Cl^- dependent co-transport of ions and catecholamines. Energy for this is derived from Na^+–K^+ ATPase and so uptake is inhibited by ouabain.

Synaptic uptake transporters for NA, DA, 5-HT, glutamate and GABA are glycoproteins with 12 transmembrane domains. Neuronal NA uptake is by uptake 1 and that into extra-neuronal tissues is by uptake 2. The two mechanisms differ.

Synaptic catecholamine uptake inhibitors:

> **amphetamine**
> **cocaine***
> **mazindol***†
> **methylphenidate**†
> **tricyclic antidepressants**†
> * also 5-HT transporter uptake inhibitors.
> † greater activity at NA uptake transporter than DA transporter.

Catecholamine catabolism: involves two main enzymes: **monoamine oxidase (MAO)** and **catechol-O-methyltransferase (COMT)**.

MAO is found in the outer membrane of *m*itochondria in both neurones and glial cells. Also found in liver and kidney cells. Requires flavin adenine dinulcleotide (FAD) as cofactor and catalyses oxidative deamination of monoamines.

Two types:

	MAO-A	**MAO-B**
preferred substrates	NA, Ad, DA, 5-HT	β-Phenylethylamine, benzylamine, DA

MAO-B is found in platelets and its level is stable with time, though there is a tendency for these to increase with age.

MAO inhibitors

irreversible	non-selective	**isocarboxacid**	
		pargyline	
		tranylcypromine	
	selective	**clorgyline**	(MAO-A)
		deprenyl	(MAO-B)
reversible	selective	**moclobemide**	(MAO-A)

*C*OMT is found in the synaptic *c*left. It exists in both soluble and membrane-bound forms and it is also found in liver, kidney and heart cells. Brain COMT in soluble form is largely extra-neuronal (glial cells, ependymal cells, cells of choroid plexus).

The enzyme is Mg^{2+}-dependent and catalyses the transfer of a methyl group from S-adenosyl-methionine (SAM) to a hydroxyl group of catechol compounds.

COMT is inhibited by   **pyrogallol** and **tropolone.**

Serotonin

Serotonin synthesis Serotonin is an indolealkylamine (5-hydroxy-tryptamine, 5-HT) neurotransmitter synthesized from tryptophan. The rate-limiting step in synthesis is catalysed by **tryptophan hydroxylase** (TrpH). This enzyme is specific to serotonergic neurones and therefore can also serve as a marker for 5-HT neurones.

TrpH is synthesized in the cell bodies and transported to the nerve terminals. It can be inhibited by **p-chlorophenylalanine** (PCPA), 6-fluorotryptophan and **p-chloroamphetamine** (PCA).

Central serotonergic nuclei

N.raphe pallidus   N. raphe dorsalis
N. raphe obscuris   N. raphe pontis
N. raphe magnus   N. raphe centralis superior

Serotonin storage and release (see Figure 11.4) 5-HT is stored in vesicles bound to serotonin-binding protein (SBP). It is released into the synapse following membrane depolarization induced calcium influx and exocytosis. **Fenfluramine** and **PCA** release serotonin.

Release is regulated by somatodendritic (5-HT_{1A}) and pre-synaptic (5-HT_{1B} and 5-HT_{1B}) autoreceptors that inhibit cell firing and 5-HT release respectively. Autoreceptor antagonists such as **pindolol** can therefore augment 5-HT release.

Serotonin inactivation

Serotonin uptake A carrier-mediated energy-dependent process. The 5-HT transporter belongs to a family of carrier proteins and has 12 transmembrane domains. 5-HT binds to the carrier in protonated form (5-HT^+) and is co-transported, with Na^+ and Cl^- ions, across the membrane and then returns bound to K^+.

Serotonin uptake is inhibited by tricyclic antidepressants (TCAs) such as imipramine and clomipramine and more selectively by 'selective serotonin re-uptake inhibitors' (SSRIs) such as citalopram, fluoxetine, fluvoxamine, paroxetine and sertraline. Inhibition of synaptic re-uptake increases the synaptic concentration of 5-HT.

Serotonin metabolism MAO metabolizes 5-HT by oxidative deamination. The resulting aldehyde is oxidized to 5-hydroxyindoleacetic acid (5-HIAA). 5-HIAA diffuses out of neurones into cerebrospinal fluid (CSF). 5-HIAA is removed from the CSF by the choroid plexus and this process is inhibited by **probenecid**.

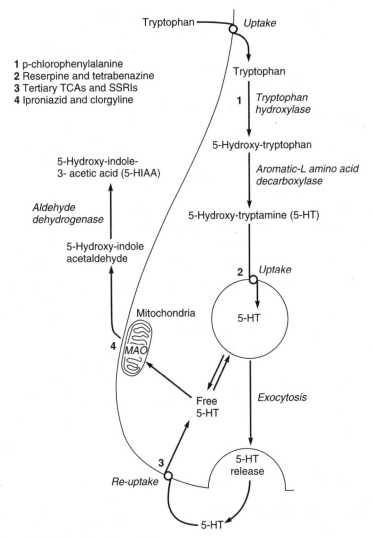

Figure 11.4 *Serotonergic neurone*

Excitatory amino acids (Eaa)

Amino acid (aa): consists of an α-carbon atom that has four different chemical groups attached to it (exception glycine). Hence two stereoselective isomers denoted L and D forms. L is aa's predominant form *in vivo*. At physiological pH aa's are ionized and possess both negative and positive charges and therefore known as **zwitterions**. If an aa side-chain has an amine group then it is likely to be a basic aa; if the side-chain has a carboxyl group then it is likely to be an acidic aa.

EAAs: Glutamate is the principal EAA. Additionally there is some evidence supporting a similar more limited role for aspartate and possibly others such as cysteic acid and homocysteic acid.

Glutamate

Glutamate is a non-essential aa that is synthesized by α-ketoglutarate (AKG) transamination. The enzyme alanine aminotransferase has pyridoxal phosphate as a cofactor and AKG is derived from the oxidative metabolism of glucose (glycolysis).

Glutamate is also synthesized from glutamine. Glutamine is stored in astrocytes and an ATP requiring mitochondrial enzyme, glutaminase, converts glutamine to glutamate.

$$\text{glutamine} + H_2O + ATP \rightarrow \text{glutamate} + ADP + NH_4^+ + PO_4^-$$

This reaction forms part of the glutamine cycle. In this glutamine is synthesized from glutamate catalysed by glutamine synthetase. There is differential localization of substrates and enzymes in neuronal endings and neighbouring astrocyte processes.

Breakdown of glutamate can be by conversion to glutamine (as described), by transamination to AKG or by oxidative deamination to AKG by glutamate dehydrogenase.

Glutamate is found in the hippocampus, its projections and those of neocortical pyramidal cells and also in cerebellar cortical parallel fibres. However, accurate functional localization is difficult because glutamate is precursor to GABA and is an intermediary in metabolic processes.

Inhibitory amino acids (GABA and glycine)

Gamma-aminobutyric acid (GABA) GABA is widely distributed within the brain and is synthesized via a single reaction catalysed by glutamate decarboxylase. This enzyme which has pyridoxal phosphate as a cofactor converts L-glutamate to GABA within neuronal axon terminals.

GABA is metabolized by a mitochondrial enzyme, GABA aminotransferase, which converts it along with AKG to glutamate and succinic semialdehyde. The latter is converted to succinate and the metabolism of AKG to succinate in this manner is called the 'GABA shunt'.

- **allylglycine:** inhibits glutamate decarboxylase
- **Gamma-vinyl GABA (vigabatrin)** inhibits GABA aminotransferase.

Synaptic release of GABA from vesicular storage is by exocytosis and re-uptake is via GABA transporters, of which there are two types. Uptake can be inhibited by **nipecotic acid, β-alanine** and **2,4,diaminobutyric acid (DABA).**

Glycine Glycine is synthesized from serine in a single reaction catalysed by serine hydroxymethyltransferase which has tetrahydrofolate as a cofactor. It can also be synthesized by the transamination of glyoxylate derived from glycolysis or the TCA cycle. Glycine is metabolized to glutathione or guanidoacetic acid.

Synaptic release is by exocytosis and uptake is via sodium dependent transporters of which there are three types (GlyT-1a, GlyT-1b and GlyT-2). GlyT-1a and 1b are found predominantly in grey and white matter respectively while GlyT-2 is found in the cerebellum, brain stem and spinal cord. Spinal cord Renshaw cell motor neurone inhibition is glycine mediated and it plays an important role in both motor and sensory systems.

Histamine Histamine is a biogenic amine that is synthesized from histidine by decarboxylation (histidine decarboxylase). Peripherally it is found in mast cells and takes part in many inflammatory and allergic reactions. Histamine is found in the brain in histaminergic neurone cell bodies, situated mainly in the hypothalamus, mast cells, neurolipomasto-cytes and capillary endothelial cells. Histamine is often co-localized with GABA or neuropeptides. Following synaptic release there is no uptake and instead histamine is inactivated by enzymes histamine N-methyltransferase and MAO-B.

Receptors All recognized neurotransmitters have been found to have more than one type of receptor (receptor subtypes).

Receptor subtypes may be derived from common genes through gene duplication, mutation and recombination or via alternative mRNA splicing. Receptor subtypes confer neurotransmitters diversity of effect (e.g. excitation/inhibition through differing transduction mechanisms) and can be characterized pharmacologically and through gene cloning.

Neurotransmitter receptors (NtRs) belong to one of two families of membrane proteins:

1 **G-protein-coupled neurotransmitter receptors** (GP-NtRs) **(metab-otropic receptors)** (action reliant on metabolic steps): consist of a single protein molecule with seven transmembrane regions (domains). Four of these domains form part of the extracellular NT binding site and two intracellular regions of the protein form the G-protein binding

site. GP-NtRs are coupled to specific **G-proteins** which, once activated, stimulate membrane effectors. These are usually enzymes involved in **second messenger systems** which in turn mediate cellular responses. These types of NtRs are relatively slow to respond.

2 **Ligand-gated channels (ionotropic receptors)**: consist of five subunits arranged in the membrane to provide an ion channel. The channel possesses an NT binding site which acts as a gate. Subunit heterogeneity provides functional variety through differential specificity of different subunits. The ionic permeability of the channel determines its action. Receptor function can be further modulated through occupancy of **allosteric binding sites**. These types of NtRs are fast acting.

G-proteins

Heterotrimers consisting of three subunits α, β and γ. There are several different kinds of each type of subunit (e.g. α_s, α_i, α_o, α_q). α subunits have a guanyl binding site (GBS) for guanyl nucleotides (GDP and GTP) and determine overall G-protein specificity and designation (e.g. G_s proteins contain α_s subunits). G-proteins can only assume two functional conformations; GDP bound or GTP bound. When the G-protein is inactive GDP is bound to its GBS and all three subunits are associated forming a trimer. Agonist stimulated receptor interaction leads to GTP substitution of GDP and α subunit dissociation leaves behind a $\beta\gamma$ dimer. The α subunit and $\beta\gamma$ dimer are then able to activate further effectors until the α subunit acting as a GTPase mediates GTP hydrolysis (to GDP) resulting in its re-association with the $\beta\gamma$ dimer. This then is the cycle of G-protein function.

Table 11.1 G-protein second messenger

G-protein	Second messenger system activation	Sensitivity to toxins (cholera/pertussis)
G_s	↑ adenyl cyclase/cAMP	Cholera
G_i	↑ adenyl cyclase/cAMP	Pertussis
G_o	Direct action on ion channels	Pertussis
$G_{t\,(transducin)}$	↑ cGMP phosphodiesterase (retinal cones/rods)	Both
G_q	↑ phospholipidase C (phophoinositide messenger system)	Neither

Second messenger systems

Three major second messenger systems:

1 **Adenylyl cyclase/cAMP system**: the membrane glycoprotein adenylyl cyclase contains two cytoplasmic catalytic domains and 12 transmembrane regions. Stimulation by the G_s-α subunit activates adenylyl cyclase which converts ATP to cAMP (Mg^{2+}-dependent process). In some instance cAMP binds directly to ion channels; however, in most cases cAMP activates protein kinases. Protein kinase A (PKA) consists of two catalytic and two regulatory subunits. When two molecules of cAMP bind to the regulatory subunits the catalytic subunits are released and can phosphorylate proteins.

2 **Phosphoinositide system**: the membrane phospholipid phosphatidylinositol 4,5-bisphosphate (**PIP_2**) is subject to hydrolysis by two forms of phospholipase C (**PLC**) (one form is G-protein coupled the other is associated with neurotrophin-sensitive protein tyrosine kinase receptors). PIP_2 hydrolysis produces two second messengers, inositol triphosphate (**IP_3**) and diacylglycerol (**DAG**). The latter remains in the membrane and stimulates protein kinase C (**PKC**). IP_3 diffuses into the cytoplasm and binds to a specific endoplasmic reticulum (ER) receptor to release Ca^{2+}. Ca^{2+} then interacts with **calmodulin** (Ca^{2+} binding protein) to form a complex (CaM) which modulates the activity of several proteins (some types of adenylyl cyclase, cytoskeletal proteins tau and MAP-2, and kinases, particularly CaM dependent protein kinase II).

3 **Arachidonic acid (AA)/phospholipase A_2 system**: membrane phospholipids contain an unsaturated fatty acid arachidonic acid (AA) which can be released by the action of phospholipase A_2. AA can be metabolized to a variety of eicosanoids that act as messengers. AA is metabolized by the following:

lipoxygenase	$\Rightarrow$	**leukotrienes**
cyclooxygenase	$\Rightarrow$	**prostaglandins** and thromboxanes
cytochrome P-450	$\Rightarrow$	epoxy-eicosatrienoic acid
autooxidation	$\Rightarrow$	hydroperoxy acid

Acetylcholine receptors

Some effects of ACh are mimicked by muscarine and others by nicotine. Muscarine and nicotine are both alkaloids (bitter tasting, nitrogen containing substances usually derived from plants) and are found in amanita muscaria (fly agaric mushroom) and nicotania tabacum (tobacco plant) respectively. Hence muscarinic and nicotinic receptors.

Nicotinic receptors: ligand-gated ionotropic receptors with rapid responses (ms) that are always excitatory. The membrane spanning pentameric neuronal nicotinic receptor contains a central cation conducting pore of 0.65 nm diameter. It is made up of five glycoprotein subunits and two of these (designated α subunits) bind an ACh molecule each. Channel opening requires both α subunit sites be occupied and this is facilitated by positive cooperativity. Intrinsic to this receptor is the ability to undergo desensitization.

Nicotinic receptors are found in striated muscles, postganglionic neurones (sympathetic and parasympathetic*) and chromaffin cells* of adrenal medulla. (*Also have muscarinic receptors.)

Muscarinic receptors: G-protein coupled metabotropic receptors with slower responses that can be either excitatory or inhibitory. Five subtypes of muscarinic receptors M1–5. Muscarinic receptors are found in cardiac and smooth muscle with parasympathetic innervation, in sweat, salivary and tear glands.

Receptor subtype actions	M2 and M4	inhibit adenylyl cyclase (striatum)
	M1, M3 and M5	release IP_3 and DAG increase cAMP arachidonic acid metabolism (hindbrain; cerebellum)
Cholinergic agonists:	**carbachol** and **methacholine** (resistant to cholinesterase degradation and do not cross BBB)	
Nicotinic agonists:	**nicotine** and **methylcarbachol** **succinylcholine** and **decamethonium** (muscle receptor depolarization block, no central effects)	
Nicotinic antagonists:	**hexamethonium** and **mecamylamine** (affinity for ganglia) **d-tubocurarine** and **gallamine** (affinity for muscle, no central effects)	
Muscarinic agonists:	**muscarine** and **pilocarpine** and **arecoline**	
Muscarinic antagonists:	**atropine** and **scopolamine** M1-**pirenzepine**	

Dopamine receptors

G-protein coupled and designated D1–5. D2 has two isoforms. Receptors fall into two groups: D1-like (D1 and D5) and D2-like (D2, D3 and D4).

D1-like linked via Gs to adenylate cyclase; D2-like negatively coupled via Gi to adenylate cyclase.

D1, D2 and D3 receptors are abundant in the nucleus accumbens, and olfactory tubercles. Additionally D1 and D2 also have a rich presence in the caudate and putamen (D2 > D1) and D3 is predominant in limbic areas and the hypothalamus.

D4 receptors have a high concentration in the frontal cortex, brain stem, and diencephalon while D5 receptors are more localized to the hippocampus and hypothalamus. Only D2 and D4 receptors have significant presence in the pituitary and the genes for these receptors are both carried on chromosome 11. D2-like receptors (D2, D3, D4) have both pre- and post-synaptic functions. As autoreceptors they can diminish cell firing and inhibit DA synthesis/release. D1-like receptors have only post-synaptic functions.

Many DA receptor binding drugs show little selectivity. Compounds with some selectivity, however those that do are:

- D1 receptor agonists: **SKF 38393**
- D2 receptor agonists: **bromocriptine; apomorphine**
- D2 receptor antagonists: **haloperidol: sulpiride; raclopride; pimozide; spiperone; domperidone**
- D3 receptor agonists: **pergolide; quinpirole; 7-OH-DPAT.**

Adrenoceptors

G-protein coupled receptors sensitive to noradrenaline and adrenaline.

Defined as α or β adrenoceptors on basis of agonist potency:

- α adrenoceptor: NA~Ad > isoprenaline (antagonized by phentolamine)
- β adrenoceptor: isoprenaline > Ad~NA (antagonized by propranolol).

Agonists/antagonists further distinguish:

- α adrenoceptors: α_1 and α_2
- β adrenoceptors: β_1, β_2 and β_3.

α_1 adrenoceptors are excitatory and post-synaptic. They are involved in smooth muscle contraction and glandular secretion.

α_2 adrenoceptors are inhibitory and both post- and pre-synaptic. Found in brain.

β_1 adrenoceptors are found mainly in heart tissue and within brain neurones.

β_2 adrenoceptors are more localized to glia and blood vessels.

Table 11.2 Adrenoceptors

Adrenoceptor	Agonist	Antagonist	Second messenger
α_1	Phenylephrine Methoxamine	Prazosin Phenoxybenzamine	Ca^{2+} DAG and IP_3
α_2	Clonidine	Yohimbine	$\downarrow$ cAMP
β_1	Dobutamine Ad = NA	Metoprolol	$\uparrow$ cAMP
β_2	Salbutamol Ad $\gg$ NA	Butoxamine	$\uparrow$ cAMP

Serotonin receptors

Four established classes of receptor: $5\text{-}HT_1$, $5\text{-}HT_2$, $5\text{-}HT_3$ and $5\text{-}HT_4$.

$5\text{-}HT_1$ receptors are further subdivided into $5\text{-}HT_{1A}$, $5\text{-}HT_{1B}$ and $5\text{-}HT_{1D}$ receptors and $5\text{-}HT_2$ receptors are subdivided into $5\text{-}HT_{2A}$, $5\text{-}HT_{2B}$ and $5\text{-}HT_{2C}$ receptors. (NB $5\text{-}HT_{2C}$ receptor was previously called $5\text{-}HT_{1C}$; hence no $5\text{-}HT_{1C}$ receptor.)

Serotonin receptors can be divided according to their second messenger systems:

- $5\text{-}HT_3$ is an ionotropic ligand gated channel and is the exception
- $5\text{-}HT_{1A}$, $5\text{-}HT_{1B}$, $5\text{-}HT_{1D}$ and $5\text{-}HT_4$ receptors are G-protein linked to adenylate cyclase.
- $5\text{-}HT_{2A}$, $5\text{-}HT_{2B}$ and $5\text{-}HT_{2C}$ receptors are coupled to the phosphatidyl inositol system.

Receptor actions: (animal and human data) $5\text{-}HT_1$ – pre-synaptic receptor mediates anxiolytic responses and causes hyperphagia.

$5\text{-}HT_{1A}$ – post-synaptic receptor (animal studies) mediates hypothermia and ACTH release.

$5\text{-}HT_{1B}$ – functions as autoreceptor and possibly also as heteroreceptor on ACh, glutamate and dopamine neurones.

$5\text{-}HT_{1D}$ – functions as autoreceptor; inhibitory heteroreceptor function on trigeminal nerve terminal neuropeptide release.

$5\text{-}HT_{2A}$ – mediates increased capillary permeability, platelet aggregation, contraction of smooth muscle (blood vessels, gut, urinary tract and uterus). Located in basal ganglia, cortex and claustrum and may mediate hallucinogenic effect of LSD.

Table 11.3 Serotonin receptors

Receptor	Agonist	Antagonist	High density regions
5-HT$_{1A}$	8-OH-DPAT; ipsapirone; buspirone	Pindolol; cyanopindolol; spiroxatrine	Hippocampus (CA1); raphe nuclei
5-HT$_{1B}$	Sumatriptan	Pindolol; isamoltane	Globus pallidus; substantia nigra
5-HT$_{1D}$	Sumatriptan	Metergoline	Basal ganglia
5-HT$_{2A}$	alpha-methyl 5-HT	Ketanserin; spiperone	Cerebral cortex (layer IV)
5-HT$_{2B}$	alpha-methyl 5-HT	Rauwolscine	Cerebral cortex (layer IV)
5-HT$_{2C}$	alpha-methyl 5-HT; mCPP	N-desmethylclozapine; ketanserin	Choroid plexus
5-HT$_3$	m-chlorophenyl-biguanide; 2-methyl-5-HT	Ondansetron; granisetron; tropisetron; zacopride	Entorhinal cortex; area postrema; peripheral neurones; vagus nerve nuclei
5-HT$_4$	Renzapride		Globus pallidus; substantia nigra; caudate n.

5-HT$_{2B}$ – stimulation causes mild anxiety and hyperphagia (animal studies) and vasodilatation may be precipitant of migraine.

5-HT$_{2C}$ – possibly regulates CSF production. Other functions not yet clear but probably mediates anxiety and panic.

5-HT$_3$ – wide distribution peripherally and centrally. Involved in cardiac, lung and intestinal activity, mediate vasodilatation, and stimulation causes pain, **nausea** and vomiting.

5-HT$_4$ – mediates cortisol secretion and contraction of colon and bladder. Centrally mediates striatal dopamine release.

Most serotonergic compounds act on several 5-HT receptor sub-types. Some (e.g. 5-HT$_{1A}$ and 5-HT$_{2C}$ anxiolytic and anxiogenic respectively) have opposing effects and so the role of specific receptors is not yet fully known.

Histamine receptors

Three subtypes: H$_1$, H$_2$ and H$_3$. H$_1$ and H$_2$ are coupled to G-proteins and act via phosphoinositide and adenylyl cyclase second messengers respectively.

H_1 receptors – widely distributed both peripherally and centrally. Particularly dense in hypothalamus, cerebellum and limbic system. Selective agonist: 2-thiazolylethylamine. Antagonists: diphenhydramine and mepyramine. H_1 receptor activation stimulates wakefulness and suppresses slow-wave sleep.

H_2 receptors – wide distribution in peripheral tissues and role in gastric acid secretion is of particular clinical importance. Centrally located in forebrain dopamine terminal areas such as striatum. Agonist: dimaprit. Antagonists: ranitidine and cimetidine.

H_3 receptor – autoreceptor and heteroreceptor. Agonist: methylhistamine. Antagonist: thioperamide.

Clinically, H_1 receptor blockers cause sedation. Newer drugs (terfenadine, astemizole) do not cross BBB and therefore avoid this adverse effect.

EAA receptors (glutamate receptors) (see Figure 11.5)

Glutamate receptors are functionally heterogenous and can be ionotropic (ligand-gated channels) or metabotropic (G-protein coupled).

The ionotropic receptors are further characterized according to their prototypical agonist and named accordingly. Hence:

Ionotropic glutamate receptors

– AMPA (α-amino-3-hydroxy-5-methyl-4-isoxazole propionic acid)
– NMDA (N-methyl-D-aspartate)
– kainate/kainic acid (extracted from seaweed).

Agonists with some selectivity: quisqualate (AMPA); ibotenic acid (NMDA); domoic acid (kainate).

All three ionotropic receptor channels are permeable to Na^+ and K^+ but only NMDA receptors are additionally permeable to Ca^{2+}.

AMPA and kainate receptors are central to fast excitatory transmission and give rise to fast EPSPs.

NMDA receptor EPSPs are slow and involve Ca^{2+} activation of calcium-dependent processes.

AMPA and NMDA receptors interact such that the NMDA receptor channel is sensitive to voltage-dependent blockade by Mg^{2+} ions (Magnesium ion binding site). This block can be removed by depolarization brought about by AMPA receptor activation. NMDA receptors also have an important interaction with glycine. Glycine binds to a separate site on the NMDA

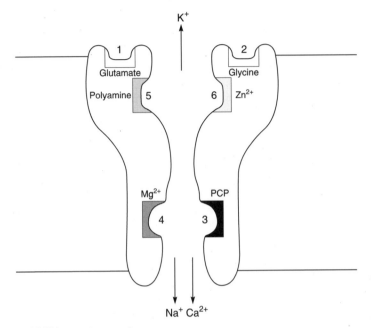

NMDA receptor complex:
1 L-glutamate binding site. Agonists promote high conductance channel opening permitting Na^+ & Ca^{2+} entry.
2 Strychnine-insensitive glycine binding site. Occupancy necessary for glutamate efficacy. Normal concentration saturates site and produces tonic stimulation.
3 Phencyclidine binding site (PCP). Also binds ketamine and dizocilpine (non-competitive antagonists). *Use-dependent blockade.*
4 Magnesium binding site (Mg^{2+}). Voltage-dependent. *Blockade.*
5 Polyamine binding site. Binds spermine and spermidine. *Facilitatory.*
6 Zinc binding site (Zn^{2+}). Voltage-independent. *Blockade.*

Figure 11.5 *NMDA receptor complex*

receptor complex (NMDA-rc) and its occupancy of this site is essential for activation of the receptor by glutamate. (NB the NMDA receptor complex glycine binding site is not sensitive to strychnine but is sensitive to the agonist D-serine.) The NMDA-rc also has other regulatory sites:

– PCP (phencyclidine) site, which also binds ketamine. These non-competitive antagonists exhibit use-dependent blockade of the channel
– polyamine site: binds spermidine and spermine (involved in tissue growth). Facilitates NMDA-rc transmission (can do both ↑↓)
– zinc ion (Zn^{2+}) binding site: voltage-independent block of NMDA-rc.

Metabotropic glutamate receptors Seven receptors (mGluR1–7) grouped according to second messenger coupling, pharmacology and aa sequence homology: (trans-ACPD is a rigid glutamate analogue that has selective agonist activity at metabotropic glutamate receptors).

- group 1: mGluR1 and mGluR5 use phosphoinositide system and are sensitive to quisqualate and trans-ACPD
- group 2: mGluR2 and mGluR3 inhibit adenylate cyclase and are sensitive only to trans-ACPD not to quisqualate
- group 3: mGluR4, mGluR6 and mGluR7 inhibit adenylate cyclase and are insensitive to both trans-ACPD and quisqualate. Group 3 receptors are instead sensitive to phosphorylated aa's and possibly function as autoreceptors inhibiting glutamate release.

Continuous neuronal stimulation by EAAs can lead to cell damage and death. This is called **excitotoxicity** and is possibly the basis of injury in epilepsy, ischaemia, amyotrophic lateral sclerosis and Huntingdon's disease.

Glutamate receptors are involved in the phenomenon of long-term potentiation (LTP), thought to be the basis of learning and memory storage.

GABA receptors (see Figure 11.6)

Three GABA receptors: $GABA_A$, $GABA_B$, $GABA_C$.

- **$GABA_A$**: ionotropic receptor (ligand-gated channel) mediating fast post-synaptic IPSPs and permeable to Cl^- ions. Can be blocked by competitive (bicuculline-binds to GABA binding site) and non-competitive (picrotoxin) antagonists producing convulsions. Benzodiazepines, barbiturates, ethanol and anaesthetic steroids potentiate the effects of GABA on $GABA_A$ receptors. The $GABA_A$ receptor consists of five glycoprotein subunits and has variety of modulatory sites.
- **$GABA_B$**: G-protein coupled receptors that are pre- and post-synaptic. $GABA_B$ receptor G-proteins interact directly with ion channels (activate K^+ channels and inhibit Ca^{2+} channels), activate phospholipase A_2, or inhibit adenylate cyclase.
  Selective agonist: baclofen and saclofen. Antagonists: 2-hydroxysaclofen and phaclofen.
- **$GABA_C$**: like $GABA_A$ receptors, form Cl^- channels but consist of novel subunits $\rho1$ and $\rho2$ (found in retina). Insensitive to bicuculline and baclofen and not affected by barbiturates or benzodiazepines.

GABA plays a crucial regulatory role and inhibits neurotransmission through both pre- and post-synaptic mechanisms.

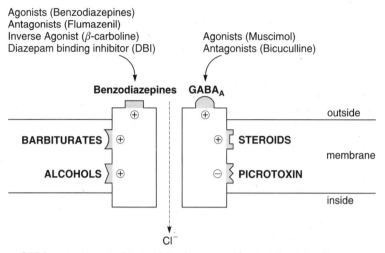

GABA$_A$ receptor complex consists of two α and β sub-units and a single γ sub-unit. Pentameric structure forms intrinsic Chloride (Cl$^-$) channel that is positively and negatively modulated by a variety of ligands and drugs

Figure 11.6   *GABA$_A$ receptor complex*

Glycine receptor

The glycine receptor is an ionotropic receptor containing a ligand-gated channel for Cl$^-$ ions which produces fast post-synaptic IPSPs. The receptor is a pentamer composed of two subunits (3α, 2β). **Strychnine**, derived from the seeds of a tree (*Strychnos nux vomica*), is a potent glycine receptor antagonist. It binds to the α subunit of the receptor causing muscle stiffness, convulsions and death.

12 *Psychopharmacology*

Antipsychotics (neuroleptics)

Typical (cause neurolepsis in experimental animals):

- **Phenothiazines:**
  - **(aliphatic side-chain):** chlorpromazine, promazine, methotrimeprazine
  - **(piperazine side-chain):** trifluoperazine, prochlorperazine, fluphenazine (depot), perphenazine
  - **(piperidine side-chain):** thioridazine, pipothiazine (depot), pericyazine.
- **Thioxanthenes:** flupenthixol (depot), zuclopenthixol (depot).
- **Butyrophenones:** haloperidol, droperidol, benperidolhaldol (depot).
- **Diphenylbutylpiperidines:** fluspirilene (depot), pimozide.
- **Substituted benzamide:** sulpiride.

Atypical (non-cataleptogenic)

- clozapine (dibenzozepine)
- risperidone (benzisoxazole derivative)
- amisulpiride (dibenzodiazepine)
- olanzapine (thienobenzodiazepine)
- sertindole (imidazoline derivative)
- quetiapine (dibenzothiazepine).

Antipsychotic effects (derived from receptor interactions)

Typical antipsychotics Act on the following:

- post-synaptic mesolimbic (ventral tegmental area [VTA] A10 → limbic system [amygdala, n. accumbens, pyriform cortex, lateral septal n.]) and mesocortical [VTA → septo-hippocampal region and frontal cortex] D2 receptor blockade: responsible for clinical antipsychotic effect.
- tuberoinfundibular system (hypothalamic arcuate n., A12 → median eminence) dopamine acts as prolactin release inhibiting factor through pituitary anterior lobe mammotroph D2 receptors: blockade causes hyperprolactinaemia – galactorrhoea, gynaecomastia, amenorrhoea, impotence, infertility.

– nigrostriatal system (substantia nigra pars compacta, A9 → striatum)
D2 receptor blockade causes extrapyramidal signs and symptoms –
parkinsonism, akathisia, tardive dyskinesia, dystonia.
– α_1-adrenoceptors: blockade causes orthostatic hypotension, dizziness,
reflux tachycardia and ejaculatory failure.
– M_1-muscarinic receptors: central blockade – seizures and pyrexia;
peripheral blockade – blurred vision, urinary retention, constipation,
sinus tachycardia, amnesia and reduced secretions (dry mouth).
– H_1-histamine receptors: blockade results in sedation, weight gain and
possibly anti-emetic effect via action on chemosensitive trigger zone
(CTZ).
– SHT2 receptors: blockade causes sexual disturbance (2a) and weight
gain (2c).
– endocrine systems: increased release of melanocyte stimulating
hormone (MSH), decreased secretion of antidiuretic hormone
(ADH), adrenocorticotrophic hormone (ACTH) and possibly
growth hormone.

Additional effects of typical antipsychotics

– Hypothermia (occasionally pyrexia) because of dose-related interference with temperature homeostasis.
– Photosensitivity and allergic dermatitis reactions (urticarial, oedema-
tous, petechial and maculopapular) occur early in treatment and
more so with low potency drugs e.g. chlorpromazine. Chlorpromazine can also discolour the skin especially upon exposure to the sun.
– Haematological effects: leukopaenia, agranulocytosis (incidence of
1:500 000, more likely with chlorpromazine and thioridazine),
thrombocytopaenia, haemolytic anaemia and leucocytosis.
– Jaundice (incidence of 1:1000) can occur especially with chlorpromazine and also with thioridazine. Strongly associated with phenothia-
zine use.
– Irreversible pigmentation of retina (similar to retinitis pigmentosa) seen
with high-dose (>800 mg daily) thioridazine use that can lead to
blindness (even after cessation of treatment). Deposits of deposits in
lens and cornea (not associated with changes of visual acuity) and
discoloration of conjunctiva, again more so with phenothiazines.
– Neuroleptic malignant syndrome (NMS): characterized by
1 hyperthermia (>38°C oral temp)
2 marked extrapyramidal effects (at least two): muscular lead-pipe
rigidity, marked cogwheeling, oculogyric crisis, trismus, opistho-
tonus, festinant gait, sialorrhoea, retrocollis, choreiform movements, dysphagia.
3 Autonomic dysfunction (at least two): tachycardia, hypertension
(↑ diastolic >20 mmHg) or lability of blood pressure, urinary
incontinence and marked diaphoresis.

Ideally all three features should be noted, however, diagnosis is still possible if only two of above are present and in addition there is one of the following:

- clouding of consciousness, serum creatinine kinase > 1000 IU/ml or leucocytosis

NB can also have abnormal liver function tests, hyperkalaemia high creatine phasphokinase, high myoglobinuria and an increase of EEG slow waves.

- occurs within 7 days of antipsychotic treatment (28 with depot) and in association with systemic disease.

Atypical antipsychotics Have less interaction with D2 receptors and interact with the following:

- D1 and D4 dopamine receptors
- 5-HT_2, 5-HT_{2c} and 5-HT_3 receptors.

It is thought that the action of atypical antipsychotics, in particular clozapine, is dependent upon the simultaneous blockade of 5-HT_2 serotonin receptors and D2 dopamine receptors, the former facilitating blockade of the latter with less receptor occupancy.

Additional effects of atypical antipsychotics Clozapine:

- reversible neutropenia (3%)
- potentially fatal agranulocytosis (0.8%)
- marked *s*ialorrhoea, *s*edation, *s*eizures (3–5%).

Risperidone: ***RISPERIDONE***

*R*ashes
*I*nsomnia
*S*exual dysfunction and *s*edation
*P*riapism
*E*mesis
*R*hinitis
*I*ncontinence
*D*yspepsia
*O*cular disturbances
*N*eutropenia but not agranulocytosis
*E*nzyme abnormalities (liver)

Olanzapine: ↑ in *OLANZPI*

*O*edema
*L*iver enzymes
*A*ppetite
*N*eutropenia

*Z*edation (most adverse effects are mild and transient)
*P*rolactivaemia (transient)
We*I*ght gain

Sertindole: *MNOPQRS*

*M*outh dryness
*N*asal congestion
*O*edema
*P*araesthesiae
↑ *Q*T interval (withdrawn due to reports of sudden death)
*R*hinitis
*S*exual dysfunction (↓ ejaculatory volume)

Approximate doses of **oral** antipsychotics (mg) equivalent to chlorpromazine 100 mg.

(NB in the order displayed, for many, the dose doubles.)

*R*ich *P*rivate *H*ospital *Tr*usts *L*ove *C*heap *Th*erapeutic *S*ervices

*R*isperidone	0.75
*P*imozide	1.5
*H*aloperidol	2.5
*Tr*ifluoperazine	5.0
*L*oxapine	10–20
*C*lozapine	50
*Th*ioridazine	100
*S*ulpiride	200

Antipsychotic depot injections

*F*lupenthixol and *F*luphenazine decanoate can be administered relatively frequently (every 2 weeks) whereas haloperidol decanoate and pipothiazine palmitate depot treatments are usually administered 4-weekly.

Table 12.1 Comparison of routes of administration

	Advantages	Disadvantages
Oral medication	Relatively short duration of effect; allows more flexible clinical management; usually more appealing than injection	Burden on patient to remember to take medication; less compliance and open to abuse/ misuse
Depot injection	Better compliance and bioavailability; accurate knowledge of drug use and less risk of abuse; ensures regular clinical contact	Adverse effects of injections (painful/unpleasant and risk of infections); delay in onset of side-effects and more difficult to withdraw medication if necessary

Zuclopenthixol can be administered in two forms:

- zuclopenthixol acetate (Clopixol-*Ac*uphase) – *ac*ute illnesses
- zuclopenthixol *d*ecanoate (every 2 weeks) – *d*epot treatment.

Antidepressants and lithium

Tricyclic antidepressants (TCAs) or monoamine re-uptake inhibitors (MARIs)

Tricyclics have a three-ring structure. The number of methyl groups attached to the side-chain nitrogen determines whether a TCA is tertiary (two groups) or secondary (one group) amine. TCAs block the re-uptake of noradrenaline and serotonin ($2°$ amines > effect on NA re-uptake; $3°$ amines > effect on serotonin re-uptake). This is thought to be the basis of their therapeutic effect.

Effects on other receptors lead to their side-effects:

- muscarine receptors; dry mouth, blurred vision, urinary retention, constipation (less severe with $2°$ TCAs)
- histamine receptors; sedation and weight gain
- adrenoceptors; postural hypotension, sexual dysfunction.
- membrane *stab*ilization (sodium channel blockade); cardiotoxic effects (*s*yncope, *t*achycardia, *a*rrhythmias, *b*lood pressure drop) and reduction of seizure threshold. ECG shows flattened T waves, prolongation of QT interval and depression of ST segment.

Generally $3°$ amine TCAs are more potent and more sedating.

Notes on individual antidepressants:

- **Amitriptyline:** has mild analgesic properties. Can be administered intramuscularly (i.m.) and intravenously (i.v.).
- **Amoxapine:** related to antipsychotic loxapine and can cause tardive dyskinesia.
- **Clomipramine:** noted for serotonergic effect; and is indicated for use in phobic and obsessional states in addition to depression. Like amitriptyline, can be given i.m. or i.v.
- **Dothiepin:** a derivative of amitriptyline, has fewer autonomic adverse effects and is somewhat less cardiotoxic.
- **Doxepin:** a derivative of amitriptyline; because of serotonergic interaction has anxiolytic properties.
- **Imipramine:** is additionally used for nocturnal enuresis in children.
- **Lofepramine:** fewer anticholinergic and cardiotoxic effects. It is less sedating and safer in overdose than most other TCAs.

- **Maprotiline:** is a tetracyclic compound; it lowers the seizure threshold.
- **Mianserin:** is a tetracyclic compound; it shows minimal cardiotoxicity and has few anticholinergic effects. Its main adverse effect is sedation.
- **Nortriptyline:** like imipramine, can be used for nocturnal enuresis in children.
- **Protriptyline:** has very little sedative effect.
- **Trimipramine:** has very strong sedative effect.

Selective serotonin re-uptake inhibitors (SSRIs)

Therapeutic effect is thought to be based upon serotonin re-uptake inhibition.

Five SSRIs: **fluoxetine, fluvoxamine, sertraline, paroxetine** and **citalopram**. All are indicated for use in depressive illness. Additional indications are:

*F*luo*x*etine ⎫ Bulimia nervosa ⎫
*F*luvo*x*amine ⎬ (*F*ood disorder) ⎬
                                  ⎬ OCD (*x* = ocd)
*P*aro*x*etine ⎫ *P*anic disorder ⎬
Citalo*p*ram ⎭   ⎭

Most adverse effects are experienced at the beginning of the treatment period and gradually diminish.

Fluoxetine: *FLUOXETINE*

*F*ever
*L*iver function tests abnormalities
*U*rticarial and other allergic reactions
*O*rgasmic dysfunction (delay)
X-tra pyramidal side-effects
*E*cchymoses
*T*ension
*I*nsomnia
*N*ausea
*E*mesis

(NB with *approximate* increasing frequency: last four are most frequent: tension/anxiety, insomnia, nausea and vomiting.)

Sertraline and **citalopram**: adverse effects similar to fluoxetine.

Paroxetine and **fluvoxamine**: common adverse effects – nausea and vomiting, headaches, dry mouth and sedation. Paroxetine does not lower seizure threshold but does have a withdrawal syndrome.

Monoamine oxidase inhibitors (MAOIs)

Most MAOIs (**phenelzine, isocarboxacid** and **tranylcypromine**) irreversibly inhibit *both* monoamine oxidases A and B. **Moclobemide** is a *selective* MAOI that exerts reversible inhibition of MAO-A.

mocloBemide is only MAOI to contain the letter '*B*' yet is the only one that does *not* act on MAO-B

Normally, orally ingested tyramine undergoes MAO metabolism in the intestinal mucosa and the liver. MAO inhibition allows **tyramine** to enter the circulation and results in the prolonged release of noradrenaline. (NA is released by tyramine from neurones and its subsequent degradation is slowed because of MAO inhibition.) This results in sweating, headache, nausea and vomiting and a marked rise in blood pressure which can cause cerebral bleeding. It is commonly referred to as the 'cheese reaction' because cheese is particularly rich in tyramine and its ingestion produces marked adverse effects. Substances and foods that need to be avoided when consuming MAOIs are:

ABCDEFG

*A*lcohol – chianti, red wines and beer
*B*road bean pods
*C*heeses (exceptions – *C*ream and *C*ottage cheeses)
*D*rugs*
*E*xtracts of meat and yeast (Marmite, Bovril)
*F*ish, especially smoked or pickled
*G*ame

* drugs: direct and indirectly acting sympathomimetics (amphetamine, phenylpropanolamine). NB can often be found in nasal decongestants and cough mixtures.

ABCDEFGHI

*A*ntidepressants (tricyclics)
*B*arbiturates
*C*ocaine, pethidine and other narcotics
L-*D*opa
*E*phedrine
*F*enfluramine
*G*eneral anaesthetics
anti-*H*ypertensives
*I*nsulin

In addition to the many possible drug and food interactions, MAOIs have several adverse effects related to receptor/metabolic actions:

– muscarinic action causing dry mouth, sweating, blurred vision, urinary hesitancy and constipation

- sympatheticomimetic action (dose related) causing weight gain, hypertension, restlessness
- serotonergic action causing **serotonin syndrome** with SSRIs of L-tryptophan
- postural hypotension and ankle oedema
- agitation, nervousness and tremor
- paraesthesiae (hands/feet) and peripheral neuropathy because of pyridoxine deficiency
- increased appetite and weight gain
- sleep disturbance and sexual dysfunction
- jaundice and hepatocellular necrosis.

Atypical and novel antidepressants

- **Flupenthixol:** thioxanthene that has antidepressant properties at low dose.
- **Mirtazapine:** dual action antidepressant which enhances serotonergic and noradrenergic neurotransmission. Antagonist at 5-HT$_2$, 5-HT$_3$, H$_1$ and pre-synaptic α_2 receptors.
- **Nefazodone:** 5-HT$_2$ and α_1 receptor antagonist which also inhibits both serotonin and noradrenaline uptake.
- **Reboxetine:** selective noradrenaline re-uptake inhibitor. α_2 adrenoceptor antagonist.
- **Trazodone:** histaminergic and α_1 adrenoceptor antagonist. It is a serotonin re-uptake inhibitor and is noted for its sedative effect. Rarely it may cause priapism.
- **Tryptophan:** used in resistant depression as adjunct. Briefly withdrawn because of association with eosinophilia-myalgia syndrome.
- **Venlafaxine:** dual action antidepressant blocking re-uptake of both noradrenaline and serotonin. Less histaminergic, α adrenergic and cholinergic effects than TCAs. Like SSRIs, causes nausea upon commencing treatment. At high doses may cause marked hypertension in 10% of subjects.
- **Viloxazine:** noradrenaline re-uptake inhibitor with few anticholinergic effects.
- **Zimeldine:** potent selective 5-HT uptake inhibitor. Withdrawn in 1983 after association with Guillain–Barré syndrome.

Lithium

Lightest of alkali earth metals exists as monovalent cation Li$^+$. Used originally (1860s) for the treatment of gout and only more recently, almost a century later, for the treatment of mania.

Rapidly absorbed following oral ingestion reaching peak plasma levels within 2 hours. Complete absorption and distribution in total body water is achieved within 8 hours and subsequently it shifts slowly into cells. Lithium undergoes no protein binding or metabolism and is excreted unchanged in the urine.

The therapeutic plasma level is usually stated as 0.4–1.0 mmol/l.

Its mechanism of action is incompletely understood. Actions:

- reduces neurotransmitter-induced activation of second-messenger systems, probably via direct interaction with G-proteins, and thus diminishes
- adenylate cyclase production of cAMP (NB TSH stimulated T4 release is cAMP-mediated, as is the effect of ADH on nephron permeability)
- phosphoinositide metabolism
- slows neuronal repolarization via Na^+ (K^+ AT-pase)

Adverse effects of lithium:

- early effects:
    Tiredness/fatigue
    Taste (metallic)
    Thirst and hence dryness of mouth
    Tremor (particularly noticeable in hands)
- late effects:
    poor renal concentrating ability; distal convoluted tubule resistance to ADH;
    polyuria
    2° hypothyroidism leads to development of goitre
    weight gain, coarsening and loss of hair
    oedema
    cardiac arrhythmias and T-wave flattening on ECG
- toxic effects (in overdose):
    diarrhoea   dysarthria
    anorexia   ataxia
    vomiting   visual disturbances

In extreme cases toxicity (Li^+ level >2 mmol/l)

↓ Co-ordination → Confusion → Convulsions → Circulatory failure → Collapse → Coma → Corpse

Therefore it is important to monitor any changes that can lead to Dangerous toxicity:

Diuretics (thiazides)
Diarrhoea and vomiting
Dietary Deficiency of Na+ (increases renal sodium and hence lithium retention)
Dehydration

Anxiolytics

*AN*xiety is a central (brain) phenomenon involving the:

*A*mygdala (in the limbic system)
NA neurones in locus coeruleus (LC)

LC discharge is influenced by α_2 and opioid autoreceptors and serotonergic, cholinergic and GABAergic heteroreceptors.

Noradrenergic activity promotes anxiety.

Benzodiazepines

Benzodiazepines bind to neuronal membrane receptors in the cerebral cortex, midbrain and limbic structures, facilitating the effects of GABA. Three endogenous ligand candidates; β-carbolines, diazepam binding inhibitor and endozepines.

Effects of benzodiazepines: with increasing dose

ASHrAM – place of religious retreat

*A*nxiolytic → *S*edative → *H*ypnotic → *A*nticonvulsant → *M*uscle-relaxant

Adverse effects:

*D*ependence
*D*rowsiness (daytime)
*D*ysarthria
*D*iplopia
*D*isorientation (especially elderly)

additionally

d *IA* z *EP AM*

*I*v → *A*pnoea, *E*lderly → *P*ainful legs, *AM*nesia

*S*topping abruptly after development of dependence (4 weeks of treatment) may lead to withdrawal symptoms:

'*S*tress' (anxiety and restlessness)
'*S*kinny' (weight loss and diminished appetite)
'*S*trange' experiences (hyperacuity of senses, derealization and depersonalization)
'*S*adness' (depressed mood)
*S*leep disturbances (rebound insomnia, ↑ stage 2 sleep with ↓ of REM and slow wave sleep)
*S*alivation

Sweating
Sexually disinterested (reduced libido)
Shaking (tremor)
Seizures

Relatively contraindicated in depression, chronic psychosis, phobic and obsessional states and absolutely so in respiratory depression and acute pulmonary insufficiency.

Benzodiazepines potentiate the effects of:

- antidepressants
- analgesics (opioid)
- antihistamines
- alcohol
- antipsychotics (phenothiazines)

and

- Disulfiram by Decreasing its Degradation.

Other drugs also thought to act on 'benzodiazepine receptors' – zopiclone and zolpidem.

Buspirone

Partial 5-HT$_{1A}$ receptor agonist (weak D2 receptor antagonist). This is thought to be responsible for its anxiolytic effect.

Unlike benzodiazepines (ashram) does not possess sedative, hypnotic, anticonvulsant or muscle-relaxant properties.

Antiepileptic drugs

0.5% of the general population is epileptic. Treatment is mainly preventative (single seizures not treated).

With treatment 2 have > 1 seizure per month, 2 have < 1 seizure per year (remainder have frequencies in between).

Carbamazepine

An iminostilbene related to TCAs; acts by limiting the repetitive firing of sodium dependent APs. Indicated in the treatment of simple and complex partial seizures secondary to a focal discharge. (NB additional applications; mood stabilizer and treatment of trigeminal neuralgia).

Dose-related adverse effects:

- cognitive impairment
- dizziness
- diplopia
- ataxia
- headaches
- nausea and vomiting.

Effects from chronic use:

- hyponatraemia.

Hypersensitivity:

- rashes
- bone-marrow suppression.

Phenytoin

A hydantoin; acts by limiting the repetitive firing of sodium dependent APs. Useful in the treatment of all forms of epilepsy except absence seizures. It has a non-linear dose–plasma concentration relationship and a narrow therapeutic index.

Dose-related adverse effects:

- dysarthria
- sedation
- ataxia.

Effects from chronic use:

- folate deficient anaemia
- osteomalacia
- gingival hyperplasia
- facial features coarsen
- hypertrichosis
- cerebellar atrophy.

Hypersensitivity:

- rashes
- hepatitis.

Sodium valproate

Action on GABA neurotransmission. Useful in the treatment of all forms of epilepsy. Note that routine plasma concentration monitoring is unhelpful.

Dose-related adverse effects:

- irritability
- tremor
- weight gain
- intestinal irritation.

Effects from chronic use

- alopecia
- amenorrhoea.

Hypersensitivity:

- hepatotoxicity
- pancreatic failure.

Ethosuximide

Acts possibly by hindering Ca^{2+} ion movements. Drug of choice in simple absence (petit mal) seizures.

Dose-related adverse effects:

- anorexia
- sedation
- psychosis
- nausea and vomiting.

Hypersensitivity:

- bone marrow suppression (leucopenia)
- rashes.

Phenobarbitone

Acts by enhancing the effects of GABA. Can be used in all forms of epilepsy except absence seizures.

Dose-related adverse effects:

- cognitive impairment
- ataxia
- sedation.

Effects from chronic use:

- folate deficient anaemia
- osteoporosis because of inhibition of vitamin D absorption.

Hypersensitivity:

- rashes.

Vigabatrin

γ-vinyl substituted analogue of GABA; acts by inhibiting GABA aminotransferase. Indicated for use in chronic epilepsy, not satisfactorily managed by other antiepileptics, and West's syndrome (infantile spasms).

Dose-related adverse effects:

- weight gain
- sedation
- depression.

Effects from chronic use:

- ? loss of peripheral vision.

Lamotrigine

Through its action on sodium channels it inhibits the release of glutamate. It is used for partial and secondarily generalized tonic–clonic seizures and those associated with Lennox Gastaut syndrome.

Dose-related adverse effects:

- rash
- ataxia
- diplopia
- vomiting
- headache.

Hypersensitivity:

- rashes
- hepatic dysfunction.

Novel agents/adjuncts

- Acetozolamide: carbonic anhydrase inhibitor.
- Benzodiazepines: clobazam, clonazepam, diazepam.
- Gabapentin: used in the treatment of partial seizures as adjunct.
- Tiagabine: GABA re-uptake inhibitor.
- Topiramate: used in the treatment of partial seizures as adjunct.

Interactions of anti-epileptics

Plasma monitoring is particularly important when these drugs are used in combination.

Table 12.2 Effect of anti-epileptics used in combination

Effect of → on plasma levels of ↓	Carbamazepine Enzyme inducer	Phenytoin Enzyme inducer	Phenobarbitone Enzyme inducer	Sodium valproate Enzyme inhibitor
Carbamazepine		▼	▼	△
Phenytoin	▼ △		▼ △	▼ △
Ethosuximide	↓	↓		↑
Sodium valproate	▲	▼	▼	
Phenobarbitone	▲	▲		▲
Primidone	▼	▼		▲
Clonazepam	▼	▼	▼	
Lamotrigine	▼	▼	▼	▲

↑ sometimes; ▲ significant effect; △ smaller effect.
NB primidone is largely converted to phenobarbitone.

Electroconvulsive therapy (ECT)

Acutely the neurochemical effects of ECT are:

↑ activity of NA, DA and 5-HT.
↓ activity of ACh.

There are corresponding changes of enzyme activity and metabolite concentrations.

Chronic ECT application results in:

↑ 5-HT$_2$ (NB opposite to antidepressants), DA$_1$ and adenosine A$_1$ purine receptor densities.
↓ β-adrenoceptor and muscarinic receptor densities.

There is also an increase in secretion/concentrations of met-enkephalin, β-endorphin, vasopressin, ACTH and prolactin.

Miscellaneous treatments in psychiatric practice

Alcohol dependence

Disulfiram

Inhibits alcohol metabolism beyond acetaldehyde. This therefore accumulates upon ingestion of alcohol. In addition, disulfiram itself is metabolized to diethylthiocarbamate which inhibits DA-β-hydroxylase (catalyses DA → NA). This leads to NA deficiency and an increase in DA.

Disulfiram-ethanol reaction:

Vasodilatation (facial flush and drop in blood pressure)
Vomiting
Vertigo
Vision is blurred
Vicious headache
Visceral pains

Avoid use in:

Asthma
Breathing difficulties
Cardiovascular disease
Diabetes
Elderly
Fitting (epilepsy, history of seizures)
Gravid (pregnant)
Hepatic disease

Adverse effects of disulfiram:

- gastrointestinal upset
- halitosis
- impotence
- peripheral neuropathy
- malaise
- depression.

Opioid dependence

- **Methadone:** is an opioid agonist that is usually prescribed to substitute the use of heroin. It is gradually withdrawn preventing the onset of withdrawal symptoms.

- **Naltrexone:** is an opioid antagonist that blocks the euphoric effects of opioids and it is used to prevent relapse.
- **Lofexidine:** acting centrally like clonidine, it reduces sympathetic tone and offers symptomatic treatment of opioid withdrawal.

Dementia

Reversible anticholinesterase inhibitors (**donazepil** and **rivastigmine**) are used for the symptomatic treatment of mild to moderate Alzheimer's disease dementia.

Antimuscarinic drugs

These drugs (**benzhexol, benztropine,* orphenadrine** and **procyclidine***) are used in the treatment of Parkinson's disease, drug-induced extrapyramidal symptoms and parkinsonism. Note however, they are not effective in the treatment of tardive dyskinesia. They should not be prescribed routinely. (* Can also be administered i.m. or i.v. and may be used for the emergency treatment of acute drug-induced dystonic reactions.)

Psychosurgery

Only available in certain centres around the world.

It is used to treat intractable anxiety and depressive disorders and in particular obsessive–compulsive disorder.

Stereotactic procedures target the limbic system and its connections. The procedures currently available are:

1 Stereotactic subcaudate tractotomy (SST).
2 Anterior capsulotomy.
3 Cingulotomy.
4 Limbic leucotomy.

All procedures associated with operative risks (haemorrhage, infection etc.) and cause an increase in the incidence of seizures.

Miscellaneous uses of some psychotropic drugs

- Tetrabenazine: movement disorders; Huntingdon's chorea.
- Haloperidol: motor tics; Gilles de la Tourette syndrome.
- Haloperidol and chlorpromazine: intractable hiccup.
- Primidone: essential tremor.

- Pimozide, sulpiride and clonidine: Gilles de la Tourette syndrome.
- Desipramine: craving in cocaine dependence.
- Fluoxetine: premature ejaculation.

Pharmacokinetics

The dissociation constant of the drug and the pH of its solution determine the degree to which it is ionized. Un-ionized the drug is more than 10 000 times more soluble. Absorption rate is determined by aspects of the drug (e.g. solubility) and the absorption site (e.g. blood flow).

Absorption

The passage of a drug from its site of administration into blood. Can be **enteral** (oral, buccal, sublingual, rectal) or **parenteral** (intramuscular, subcutaneous, intravenous, intrathecal, topical, inhalational).

Table 12.3   Comparison of selected routes of drug administration

Route of administration and notes	Advantages	Disadvantages
Oral: absorption is mainly from small intestine by passive diffusion, pore filtration (most drugs too large) or active transport (specific)	Convenience Safety	Gastric acidity Presence of food in stomach.
Rectal: absorption from GIT is influenced by gut motility, blood flow and area of absorption	By-passes stomach/liver Useful with nausea/ vomiting Overcomes difficulty of swallowing (NB coma, seizure)	Embarrassment Inflammation with frequent use
Intramuscular: better for lipid-soluble drugs	Depot treatment (slow release) Safe route in emergencies No GIT irritation	Painful Risk of damage to nerves/vessels Risk of infection/abscess
Intravenous	Rapid onset of action Can titrate dose and response Avoids first-pass metabolism	Easy to overdose Infection, embolism, thrombosis Necrosis of tissues Injection into an artery

Distribution

Distribution of a drug between different body compartments (extracellular/intracellular) and different components (protein, lipids, water). It is dependent upon:

- solubility of the drug and its extent of protein binding
- tissue permeability factors (pH partition; fat-water partition)
- haemodynamic factors
- partitioning membranes (blood–brain barrier, placenta).

Body fluid compartments

Body water Forms 60–70% of body weight.

Plasma 5%; interstitial 15%; transcellular 2%; intracellular 35%; lipids 20% (% body weight).

Extracellular fluid (16 litres) = blood plasma (5 litres) + interstitial fluid (10 litres) + lymph.

Intracellular fluid (30 litres) = total fluid in all cells of the body.

Transcellular fluid (1 litre) = peritoneal, synovial, pleural, intraocular, cerebrospinal fluids and digestive secretions.

Volume of distribution The apparent volume of distribution (V_d) is a theoretical volume that is defined as the volume of fluid necessary to contain the total amount of a given drug (D) at a concentration equivalent to that in the plasma (C_p).

$$V_d = D/C_p$$

The duration of action of a drug is inversely proportional to its volume of distribution.

Body fat adds to the volume of distribution of a drug and the more lipid-soluble a drug the greater its volume of distribution. The volume of distribution of a drug increases with age because of a relative increase in body fat.

Protein binding Competitive reversible binding of drugs to plasma proteins is dependent upon:

- the free drug concentration
- the affinity of the drug for protein binding sites
- the protein concentration (reduced in cardiac failure, renal/hepatic disease, carcinoma, malnutrition, burns).

Blood–brain barrier (BBB) The brain contains neuronal and glial intracellular fluid; 200 ml of extracellular fluid and 110 ml of cerebrospinal fluid of which about 20 ml is intraventricular and the remainder is in the subarachnoid space. In addition there is 80 ml of intracranial blood plasma.

Blood in brain capillaries is partitioned from the extracellular fluid compartment by the BBB, which protects the brain by maintaining an exclusive environment.

The BBB comprises: (Brain → Blood) (important components *ABC*)

- glycoprotein and sialic acid neuronal surface covering
- perineuronal satellite cells (e.g. oligodendroglia)
- *A*strocyte end feet
- *B*asement membrane
- vessel wall
- *C*apillary endothelium.

Some substances readily cross the BBB – oxygen, carbon dioxide, glucose, some amino acids.

Permeability is generally dependent upon lipid solubility. Most psychotropics are lipophilic and cross easily. Some substances require specific active transport mechanisms to cross the BBB (many amino acids; NB these transport systems are strereospecific with preference for L-isomers).

The permeability of the BBB is increased by inflammation (effect of histamine or some bacterial endotoxins) and anoxia induced cerebral oedema.

The BBB is absent in some parts of the brain because of capillary vessel fenestration:

- hypothalamic regions, e.g. median eminence (allows releasing factors access to pituitary portal system)
- pineal body
- area postrema (vascularized strip of medullary tissue lying at caudal end of lateral border of 4th ventricle)
- choroid plexi
- hypophysis.

Placenta Placental barrier between maternal and fetal vascular systems also has protective function. Substances cross placental barrier by diffusion, active transport or pinocytosis. Lipid-soluble drugs cross more easily.

Metabolism (biotransformation)

Most drugs are altered chemically prior to elimination from the body. Biotransformation produces metabolites that are more easily excreted. It is less often necessary for small, highly water-soluble molecules, which may be excreted unaltered. Metabolism takes place principally in the liver but also occurs in several other tissues: *KILLS* drug activity

*K*idneys, *I*ntestine, *L*ungs, *L*ymphocytes, *S*kin

Hepatic metabolism involves non-synthetic and synthetic reactions.

- **Phase I** hepatic biotransformation involves non-synthetic reactions such as oxidation, reduction and hydrolysis. The products may be active and in general drugs that undergo non-synthetic reactions require further conjugation prior to elimination. Oxidation is the most common reaction and involves microsomal mixed-function oxidases (cytochrome p450 isoenzymes) located on smooth endoplasmic reticulum.

- **Phase II** hepatic biotransformation involves conjugation (synthetic reaction). In this there is chemical coupling of the drug and a water-soluble molecule from the body (glucuronate; glutathione; glycine; glutamine; acetate; sulphate). Conjugation with an endogenous water-soluble molecule produces a water-soluble conjugate which can then be excreted in urine or bile.

- **First-pass effect:** hepatic metabolism that occurs following gastro-intestinal absorption and passage via liver prior to entering systemic circulation. Dependent upon several factors, e.g. blood flow to the liver and altered by hepatic disease.

- **Enzyme induction:** the enzymes involved in biotransformation can be induced (increasing enzymatic activity) by the action of certain drugs; e.g. barbiturates, phenytoin, alcohol. This can affect the plasma concentration of the drug itself (auto-induction) and that of other drugs.

- **Enzyme inhibition**: produces indirect interactions which can cause adverse effects or occasionally be of benefit.

Excretion (elimination)

Most drugs and their metabolites undergo renal excretion. This is affected by: nephron function (GFR); the drug's plasma concentration; its solubility, protein-binding and molecular weight.

Excretion also occurs in: bile and faeces, saliva, sweat and milk. Biliary excretion of some substances is active and even when a substance has been excreted into the intestine it may undergo reabsorption (enter-ohepatic cycle). Elimination of drugs via breast milk is not significant quantitatively but is important with respect to potential toxic effects on a breast-feeding infant. Milk is of lower pH than plasma and can concentrate certain substances.

1⅗ *Genetics*

DNA and RNA

nucleo*S*ide = nitrogenous base (e.g. adenine) + *S*ugar (ribose or deoxyribose) only.

nucleo*T*ide = nucleoside + phospha*T*e

DNA (deoxyribonucleic acid) Large polymer found in chromosomes of cell nucleus and mitochondria. Linear backbone consists of successive 5-carbon sugar residues (deoxyribose) covalently linked by covalent $3',5'$ **phosphodiester bonds.** Four nucleotides (purines; **adenine** [A] and **guanine** [G] and pyrimidines; **cytosine** [C] and **thymine** [T]) form two strands that are arranged in a **double helix (DNA duplex).** The hydrogen bond **complementary** base-pairing between the two **anti-parallel** strands is always A-T and G-C (2 and 3 hydrogen-bonds respectively in each **base pair**) in accordance with **Chagraff's rule.** (NB Hydrogen bonds can be disrupted by changes of pH or heat.)

RNA (ribonucleic acid) Contains ribose instead of deoxyribose and uracil [U] instead of thymine.

There are several kinds of RNA: messenger RNA (**mRNA**), ribosomal RNA (**rRNA**), transfer RNA (**tRNA**) and heterogenous nuclear RNA (**hnRNA**).

DNA replication

The process of DNA synthesis commences with **helicase** unwinding the DNA duplex. DNA replication originates and takes place at a **replication fork.** Synthesis can only occur in the direction $5' \rightarrow 3'$ and therefore along one strand, designated the **leading strand**, replication occurs in the direction of movement of the replication fork. This is carried out continuously by **DNA polymerase δ.** Along the other strand, called the **lagging strand**, $5' \rightarrow 3'$ synthesis uses **DNA polymerase α** and is accomplished in stages using pieces called **Okazaki fragments** which are subsequently joined together by **DNA ligase.** The synthesis of DNA is therefore described as **semi-discontinuous.** The process of DNA replication is also described as **semi-conservative** because each strand directs the synthesis of a complementary one leading to two identical daughter DNA duplexes each of which contains an original strand. Complete DNA replication takes approximately 8 hours.

Genes

The human genome contains about 100 000 human genes.

Gene: DNA segment that encodes for a single/limited set of proteins.

Alternative forms of a given gene are termed **alleles.** Each gene has two alleles. If the two alleles are the same the individual is described as being **homozygous** in respect of this gene. If they differ then they are described as being **heterozygous** in respect of that particular gene.

A **dominant** gene expresses its effect even if only present on one chromosome.

A **recessive** gene is only expressed in those that are homozygous in respect of the gene.

Genes only form 1% of total human DNA. The remainder is thought to be involved in regulatory and supportive processes. Even within genes there is DNA that does not code for amino acids. These segments are called *in*trons (NB they remain *in*side the nucleus). **Exons** are transported into the cytoplasm and they code for amino acids (three nucleotide bases form a **codon** and denote a specific amino acid). The nuclear organelle, the spliceosome, splices exons into mRNA and removes introns from heterogenous RNA.

Gene expression

The flow of genetic information is largely unidirectional from DNA to RNA to polypeptides. This is known as the **central dogma of molecular biology**. Gene expression follows the **colinearity principle** and involves **transcription** and **translation**. Only a small proportion of the DNA is expressed, i.e. is **coding DNA**. Furthermore, only some of the RNA created by transcription is further translated into polypeptide/protein.

Transcription

Transcription proceeds $5' \rightarrow 3'$ and the initial step involves production of a complementary RNA transcript. Only one of the strands acts as a template **(template strand/antisense strand)**. The RNA transcript has the same orientation (5' → 3') and base sequence (U replaces T) as the non-template strand and so this is also called the **sense strand**. In addition to its structural and coding components (exons/introns) a typical gene (5' → 3') consists of a transcription regulatory site, a promotor region (e.g. TATA box; GC box; CAAT box) and a transcription initiation site. Transcription involves **RNA polymerases** (of which there are three different types I, II and III; most genes encode peptides and are transcribed by RNA polymerase II) and a variety of **transcription factors**.

Post-transcriptional processing involves RNA splicing, capping and polyadenylation.

- **RNA splicing:** most genes consist of coding sequences (**exons**) separated by non-coding sequences (**introns**) which are removed by endonucleolytic cleavage at specific **splice junctions** from the **primary transcript** (transcription of complete gene) by **spliceosomes**.
- **Capping:** RNA polymerase II transcripts undergo the addition of a specialized nucleotide to the 5' end of mRNA. This is thought to help RNA splicing, aid mRNA transport into the cytoplasm, protect the mRNA transcript from enzymatic degradation and facilitate ribosomal attachment. **Polyadenylation:** following transcript cleavage the mRNA 3' end is polyadenylated (~200 adenylate residues are added) 15–30 nucleotides downstream of the AAUAAA element. This is thought to add stability, aid mRNA transport into the cytoplasm and facilitate translation.

Translation

Translation is the specific ribosomal decoding of mRNA. Once transported out of the nucleus into the cytoplasm, mRNA undergoes translation by ribosomes which decipher the mRNA information and organize, with the use of tRNA, the appropriate amino acids to form the designated peptide. It is of note that mitochondria also contain ribosomes and are capable of protein synthesis.

In eukaryotes ribosomes (RNA-protein complexes) are composed of two subunits (large – 60S and smaller – 40S). The 40S subunit contains 18S rRNA and approximately 30 proteins; the 60S subunit contains 28S, 5.8S and 5S rRNA and about 50 proteins.

The mRNA sequence consists of successive **codons** (groups of three nucleotides) which specify individual amino acids. tRNA molecules with covalently bound specific amino acids mediate decoding (each tRNA molecule is bound to a single specific amino acid by an amino-acyl-tRNA-synthetase). Each tRNA has a specifically sited trinucleotide sequence (the **anticodon**) that interprets the genetic code and it is essential that this is recognized by the codon and that complementary base-pairing takes place between the two. In this manner a specific amino acid is inserted into the growing peptide chain. In most cases the first **initiation codon** (AUG), which specifies methionine, initiates translation. As subsequent amino acids are added, **peptidyl transferase** (within 60S ribosomal subunit) catalyses a condensation reaction (between amino group of amino acid being added and carboxyl group of amino acid in chain) which results in successive peptide bonds. Linear translation of the mRNA continues until a **termination codon** is encountered. The genetic code is described as being **degenerate** as there are many more codons than amino acids and many amino acids are specified by several codons, however, some amino acids are only specified by a single codon, e.g. tryptophan or methionine.

The initial translation product often undergoes **post-translational modification**. This includes the addition of groups (methylation (CH_3), phosphorylation (PO_4^-), hydroxylation (OH), carboxylation (COOH), acetylation (CH_3CO) and glycosylation) and internal cleavage. Many polypeptides are synthesized as precursors containing an N-terminal **signal/leader sequence**. This is usually necessary for transmembrane transport of the polypeptide.

Chromosomes

Human somatic cell nuclei contain **46** chromosomes; 22 pairs of **autosomal chromosomes** (44 autosomes) and one pair of **sex chromosomes**. Similar autosomes are paired and termed **homologous**, however, they are not identical.

Specialized sex cells (**gametes**) have half the number of chromosomes (23) and are termed **haploid** as opposed to somatic cells which are described as **diploid**. A normal male is therefore 46XY and a normal female 46XX.

Gametes arise from specific gonadal somatic cells which undergo reductive cell division termed **meiosis**. The fusion of two haploid cells produces diploid somatic cells, as indeed does binary cell division, which includes **mitosis** (nuclear division) and **cytokinesis** (cytoplasmic division).

Differentiation of somatic cells can alter their DNA content and some have no chromosomes at all (platelets, red blood cells) whereas others are multinucleated (muscle cells). Additional DNA duplication prior to cell division (**endomitosis**) results in **polypoid** cells which have additional sets of chromosomes (hepatocytes, megakaryocytes).

Chromatin The basic material of chromosomes, consisting of DNA complexed with proteins. DNA is tightly packaged to form **nucleosomes**

which consist of a central core of **histone proteins** around which 146 base-pairs of double stranded DNA are coiled. Successive nucleosomes are linked by spacer DNA and the nucleosomes themselves are further coiled to form a **chromatin fibre**. Chromatids consist of coiled loop-scaffold complexes. In these chromatin fibre loops are attached to a central scaffold protein such as topoisomerase II.

CRs are normally very thin and drawn out. Therefore they are usually examined during mitosis or meiosis when more condensed.

Karyotype

Ordered display of CRs. Preparation involves:

– cell division arrest, dispersion, fixing and staining of CRs
– CRs are then photographed and arranged according to their identity.

Number of X CRs in somatic cell nucleus can be determined without karyotyping. The number of **chromatin bodies** (**Barr bodies**, BB) equals the number of X CRs minus one. (Chromatin body number = No. of X CRs – 1; e.g. XX female = 1 BB.)

Each CR has a constricted region that is prominent during mitosis and meiosis. This is called the **centromere** and it divides CRs into two arms of differing lengths.

The long arm is designated **q,** the short arm is designated **p**.

The positioning of the centromere gives rise to **metacentric** CRs (centromere central) and **acrocentric** CRs (centromere nearer one end).

The staining of CRs produces bands that are then ascribed names and numbers. This produces a **chromosomal map**.

Standardized designation: e.g. **Xq28**

First character	(**X**)	can be letter (X or Y) or number (1–22) specifying the CR
Second character	(**q**)	specifies short or long CR arm (p or q)
Third character	(**2**)	designates particular CR region
Fourth character	(**8**)	identifies band

Cell division

In the cell cycle cell division, i.e. *mi*tosis (*M* phase), is a relatively short stage which alternates with **interphase**. Interphase is a much longer period and consists of three phases: a gap between the M and S phases

(**G1** phase), the *s* phase itself, during which DNA is *S*ynthesized, and another subsequent the gap (**G2** phase) between the S and M phase to complete the cycle. Cells that are non-dividing remain in stage G0 (a modification of G1) and only those cells that are committed to cell division enter the S phase.

Mitosis

Somatic cell nuclear division: five phases: *DIPloMAT*

*D*ivision =
*I*nterphase
*P*rophase
*M*etaphase
*A*naphase
*T*elophase

Meiosis

Reproductive cells undergo two stages of cell division resulting in haploid gametes. The stages of mitosis are repeated with exception of interphase.

Inheritance

Patterns of inheritance are best considered with examples.

Genotype: capital letter denotes dominant allele, lower case denotes recessive allele.

Gregor Mendel, Austrian monk and botanist: Mendelian inheritance applies to single gene defects (deletions, inversions, insertions).

Table 13.1   Mendelian inheritance

Parents	$DDDD \times dddd$	$DDdd \times DDdd$	$DDMM \times ddmm$
Offspring (F_1)	Dd	DD:Dd:Dd:dd	DdMm
Offspring (F_2)			DDMM, DDMm, ddmm etc.
Law of ...	Uniformity	Segregation	Independent Assortment
Mendel's		First Law	Second Law

Inheritance of disease

Autosomal dominant Dominant allele leads to manifestation of disease in all individuals that possess it. Hence shows 'vertical' transmission as phenotypic trait is evident in every generation. Affects both sexes and can be transmitted between males. Degree of penetrance and expressivity cause variance of clinical features. Spontaneous occurrence of autosomal dominant disorder may be because of a new mutation.

Autosomal recessive Expression of disease requires that individual carries two alleles (i.e. is homozygous). Heterozygous individuals carry but do not phenotypically manifest the disease and hence the disease seems to miss generations and give the appearance of horizontal transmission. Rare disorders increase the likelihood of consanguineous parents.

X-linked disorders Affected allele on X chromosome. Transmission between males is not possible. Can be **dominant** (affected allele is dominant) or **recessive** (affected allele is recessive and all males with affected allele manifest the disorder. Females if heterozygous are carriers).

Genetic studies

Conventional methods

Family, twin and adoption studies.

Family studies Comparison of the rates of a disorder in proband's relatives (first and second degree) and the general population. First degree relatives (biological parents, siblings and offspring) share 50% of genome. Second degree relatives (grandparents, uncles, aunts, nieces, nephews and grandchildren) share 25% of genome.

Disadvantages:

- common environment (hence need for twin/adoption studies)
- varying ages of relatives. Disease may not have yet presented.

(Clinically, increased incidence/prevalence is seen in relatives of those with *a*nxiety neurosis, *a*norexia nervosa, *a*lcoholism, *A*lzheimer's disease, and *a*utistic disorder.)

Twin studies Comparison of rates of a disorder in co-twins of probands (monozygotic versus dizygotic). Monozygotic twins are identical and have same genome. Dizygotic twins share 50% of genome (siblings).

Concordance rate: concurrence rate of disorder in proband co-twin.

Can be derived according to pairs (concordant sets of twins/total no. of twin sets) or probands (proband co-twins with concurrent disorder/total no. of co-twins).

Concordance rate is generally more suitable when examining discrete traits whilst correlation coefficient is better for continuous traits.

Disadvantages:

- assortative mating ($\uparrow$ in rate of illness in dizygotic twins relative to monozygotic twins)
- age correction measures and sampling may introduce bias
- twins more susceptible to injury at birth and more likely to have congenital abnormalities.

Within twins, monozygotic twins more at risk.

Adoption studies Individual is adopted away from biological parents and reared by unrelated adoptive parents. Known as **adoptee** studies.

Studies can centre on the adoptee or the whole adoptee family and can also use monozygotic twin adoptees to enhance their power. Cross-fostering is a complicated method that is occasionally used (children adopted from affected biological parents and their adoptive parents are compared with the children of unaffected biological parents and affected adoptive parents). If the rate of disorder in parents is studied, this is known as an adoptee family study.

Disadvantages:

- time consuming to conduct
- difficult to find appropriate cases (criteria difficult to fulfil)
- adoption process is not necessarily random
- data concerning biological parents may not be available
- confounding psychological influence of being adopted.

Modern methods

Meiotic **recombination** (cross-over) takes place in prophase I, allowing the exchange of genetic material between homologous chromosome pairs, altering the alleles carried. Genes that are close together are less likely to be separated during this process than those that are distant from each other. Genes that are in close proximity and are usually inherited together are described as being genetically linked. Any two genes that recombine only 1% of the time and are otherwise inherited together are described as being separated by a distance of 1 centimorgan (1 cM) along the chromosome. (1 cM is approximately 1×10^6 DNA base pairs.)

The **recombinant fraction** (RF), designated θ, is a measure of the frequency with which recombination occurs between two genes such that alleles at these loci are separated during meiotic recombination. It is expressed as a fraction, 0–0.5, or percentage, 0–50%. Concurrent inheritance with no recombination gives a recombinant fraction of zero. If genes are widely separated and independently inherited the recombinant fraction is 0.5.

The **odds ratio** is a ratio of two probabilities; that of there being linkage for a particular recombinant fraction and that of there being no linkage (i.e. any apparent co-segregation is because of linkage as opposed to chance). The logarithm of this ratio (base 10) is defined as the **lod score** (Lod score of Morton). A lod score of –2 or less excludes linkage and a score of 3 or more is taken as evidence of linkage (single-gene mendelian inheritance).

Restriction endonucleases are enzymes that selectively cleave DNA. Acting at specific nucleotide sequences they produce many small DNA fragments which form a characteristic pattern. Though consistent in a particular person the fragment pattern differs between people. This unique pattern of DNA fragments can be identified using **Southern blotting** and certain DNA probes. Polymorphisms at cleavage sites result in fragments of varying length called **restriction fragment length polymorphisms** (RFLPs). These undergo Mendelian inheritance and can be used as DNA markers. **Gene probes** are DNA pieces produced with complementary nucleotide sequences that enable them to hybridize with specific portions of the genome.

Linkage analysis uses DNA markers such as RFLPs to find an association between them and a particular disease or illness locus. If there is a departure from independent assortment (co-segregation) then linkage is inferred.

Genetic abnormalities and birth defects

One in forty pregnancies results in the birth of a child with a congenital abnormality. The cause of most is unknown. The aetiology can be genetic, environmental or multifactorial.

- Environmental factors:
    - maternal factors (prior to and during pregnancy and at the time of birth)
    - maternal illness (e.g. diabetes)

  - infections (toxoplasmosis, rubella, cytomegalovirus, herpes)
  - medications, drugs and toxins (e.g. ethanol, heavy metals, phenytoin)
  - mechanical factors (e.g. forceps delivery)
  - radiation (X-rays)
  - pollution (air and water).
- Genetic disorders:
  - chromosomal abnormalities
  - numerical changes (increase or absence)
  - structural changes (deletions and translocation)
  - single gene abnormalities
  - autosomal (dominant and recessive)
  - sex chromosome linked (dominant and recessive).
- Multifactorial.

Chromosomal abnormalities

Disorders result from:

  - a change in the **number** of chromosomes
  - change in chromosomal **structure**; deletion/loss, addition
  - **translocation** of chromosomal material between chromosomes.

5% of foetuses have chromosomal abnormalities and of these 90% abort.

0.5% of live newborn infants have chromosomal abnormalities (autosomal: sex CRs; 2:1).

Autosomal abnormalities

Down syndrome Described by Langdon Down in 18*66*. It is a common cause of mental retardation.

Few with Down syndrome have an IQ >50, and of those with mental retardation and IQ <50 one-third have Down syndrome.

Maternal age is an important risk factor:

risk at age   *20* yr   1:*20*00
               45 yr   1:*45*

Overall incidence 1:*66*0 live births.

Usually (95% of cases) trisomy 21 arises because of meiotic non-disjunction (chromosomal separation producing a gamete with an extra chromosome).

In 4% of cases the cause is translocation of genetic material between chromosome 21 and another.

In 1% of cases only a proportion of the cells have trisomy and the remainder are normal (mosaic).

The risk of recurrence with non-disjunction is about 1%, in cases of translocation the risk is much higher.

Stigmata:

- Eyes: **BCDEF**
  Brushfield's spots
  Cataracts and conjunctivitis
  Deviation (squint)
  Epicanthic folds and ectropion
  Fissure (palpebral) upwardly slanting
- Head:
  small, brachycephalic skull with flat occiput
  small rounded ears
  high cheekbones
  large fissured tongue.
- Body: **BCDEFGH**
  Bowel disorder (Hirschsprung's disease)
  Cryptorchidism
  Duodenal atresia
  Endocardial cushion defects [40–50%]
  straight **F**ollicles (pubic hair)
  poor development of external **G**enitalia
  umbilical **H**ernia
- Hands and feet:
  single palmar crease (simian) (50%)
  clinodactyly (50%)
  abnormal dermatoglyphics
  broad hands and short stubby fingers
  short, broad feet
  large cleft between 1st and 2nd toes.
- Brain:
  epilepsy [10%]
  mental retardation
  earlier development of senile plaques
  marked ↑ P300 latency.
- General:
  hypotonia
  leukaemia (1%)
  hypothyroidism (3%)
  short stature.

Edward's syndrome (trisomy 18) 95% of fetuses abort. Main cause non-disjunction.

1:3000 live births. 30% die within one month. Maternal age effect.

Stigmata:

- mental retardation
- craniofacial abnormalities: micrognathia, prominent occiput, low-set fawn-like ears
- palmar crease, abnormal dermatoglyphics and when hand is clenched overlaps fifth and index fingers
- rocker-bottom feet
- short sternum
- cardiac and renal malformations
- males (cryptorchidism).

Patau's syndrome (trisomy 13) 1:7600 live births. Virtually all die by age 3 years (50% within one month). Maternal age effect.

Stigmata:

- cleft lip/palate
- polydactyly
- ophthalmic defects
- low-set ears.

Cri-du-chat syndrome Deletion on short arm of chromosome 5. 1:50 000 live births. More common in females than males.

Stigmata:

- mental retardation
- abnormal cry
- spasticity
- craniofacial abnormalities: microcephaly, moon faced, epicanthic folds, hypertelorism and alert expression.

Prader–Willi syndrome 1:15 000 live births. Partial deletion of long arm of chromosome 15 (chromosomal derivation usually paternal).

Stigmata: *PRADER*

*P*alpebral fissures – almond shaped
*R*ound face
*A*ngry outbursts
*D*own-turned mouth
*E*at excessively (hyperphagia)
*R*educed tone (infantile hypotonia)

Small: in height; hands and feet; testicles.

Retinoblastoma Deletion on CR 13.

Stigmata:

- bilateral retinoblastoma
- reduced IQ.

W*I*lm's tumour (renal) Deletion on CR 11.

Stigmata:

*I*Q reduced
*I*urrises are absent (aniridia)
*I*ndeterminate (ambiguous) genitalia

Sex chromosome abnormalities

Kleinfelter's syndrome Occurs 1:500. Phenotypic male has extra X chromosome(s) (maternal in 60% cases). Usually 47XXY. 15% are mosaics. Maternal age effect.

Stigmata:

- infertility (usual mode of presentation)
    small testis (<2 cm length)
    low testosterone levels
    poorly developed secondary sexual characteristics
- gynaecomastia
- variable degree of mild mental retardation (often normal)
- elongated limbs (disproportionate body).

Associations: diabetes, osteoporosis, emphysema, scoliosis, breast cancer, schizophrenia.

47XYY Occurs 1:700. Phenotypic males have extra Y chromosome because of paternal YY sperm.

Stigmata:

- very tall (body proportions normal)
- IQ slightly lower than normal.

Doubtful associations with aggression and criminality.

Extra X chromosomes XXX, XXXX etc. very mild abnormalities with a single additional X chromosome; however, with each additional X chromosome degree of mental retardation becomes more evident.

Turner's syndrome Occurs 1:2500 (female births). Diagnosed by buccal mucosal cell chromosomal analysis. XO. Barr body.

60% are 45X

Remainder are deletions of X chromosome long/short arm or mosaics.

Life-span and intelligence are normal.

Stigmata:

- short stature
- craniofacial abnormalities:
    webbed neck
    micrognathia
    low hair-line (back of head)
    downward slanting palpebral fissures
    down-turned mouth
    low-set ears
- limb and truncal abnormalities:
    lymphoedema
    cubitus valgus (wide carrying angle)
    wide separation of nipples (broad, shield-like chest)
- ovarian dysgenesis (streak ovaries): infertility
- cardiovascular defects:
    atrial septal defects
    coarctation of the aorta
    hypertension
- Hashimoto's thyroiditis.

Single gene abnormalities

Autosomal dominant disorders

- Huntingdon's disease.
- Phacomatoses (tuberose sclerosis, neurofibromatosis, Sturge–Weber syndrome, von Hippel–Lindau syndrome).
- Acrocephalosyndactyly (Apert's syndrome).
- Craniofacial dysostosis (Crouzon's syndrome).
- Mandibulofacial dysostosis (Treacher Collins' syndrome).
- Wardenburg syndrome.
- Myotonic distrophy.

Autosomal recessive disorders

Metabolic disorders

- Fat metabolism:
    Niemann-Pick disease
    Tay–Sachs disease
    Gaucher's disease.

- Protein metabolism:
  phenylketonuria
  Hartnup disease.
- Mucopolysaccharidoses:
  Hurler's syndrome
  Hunter's syndrome.
- Carbohydrate metabolism:
  galactosaemia.

Others

- Cockayne's syndrome.
- Dubowitz syndrome.
- Laurence–Moon–Bardet–Biedl syndrome.
- Seckel syndrome.
- Sjögren–Larsson syndrome.
- Smith–Lemli–Opitz syndrome.

X-linked recessive disorders

- Fragile X syndrome.
- Lesch–Nyhan syndrome.
- Hunter syndrome.
- Cerebellar ataxia.
- Oculocerebrorenal syndrome (Lowe's syndrome).
- Menke's syndrome.

X-linked dominant disorders

- Rett syndrome.
- Vitamin D resistant rickets.

Autosomal dominant disorders

Tuberose sclerosis (epiloia, Bourneville's disease) 1:40 000 live
births. *A*utosomal *d*ominant.

Stigmata:

- butterfly rash: begins in crease between cheeks and nose at very
  young age (angiofibromas)
- '*ade*noma sebaceum'
- *de*ficiency (mental retardation)
- *e*pilepsy
- s*hagre*en patches – flesh-coloured, lumbo-sacral plaque-like tumours
- *h*amartomas in lungs and kidneys

- *a*melanotic naevi – macular patches of hypopigmentation (best seen with Wood's light)
- *g*liomas
- *re*tinal phakomas.

Die usually because of heart failure or pneumonia.

Sturge–Weber syndrome (encephalofacial angiomatosis) 50% have mental retardation.

Epilepsy is common.

Intracranial angioma (parieto-occipital) – often becomes calcified.

Cutaneous naevus in distribution of trigeminal nerve (ipsilateral to angioma).

Neurofibromatosis (von Recklinghausen's disease) 1:3000 live births. A third have mental retardation.

Stigmata:

- café au lait patches (>5 abnormal)
- pigmentation (melanoma, axillary freckling)
- neural tumours
    cutaneous neurofibroma, acoustic neuroma, spinal cord nerve root
        neurofibroma (dumb bell tumour)
    plexiform neuroma
    optic nerve glioma
    meningioma
- aortic coarctation
- berry aneurysm
- obstructive cardiomyopathy
- renal artery stenosis
- diabetes insipidus
- hypospadias
- mesenteric ischaemia
- phaeochromocytoma
- pulmonary fibrosis
- scoliosis
- fibrous dysplasia of bone
- local limb gigantism.

Autosomal recessive disorders

Phenylketonuria Folling (1934). Third most common known cause of mental retardation (after Down syndrome and Fragile X syndrome). 1:14 000 live births.

Absence of phenylalanine hydroxylase. Therefore conversion of phenylalanine (Phe) to tyrosine is not possible.

Tested for using the Guthrie test (*B. subtilis* – multiplication phenylalanine-dependent). (NB test 6–14 days after birth as levels of amino acid normal at birth.)

Deficiency leads to severe mental retardation (IQ <50). This can be avoided by dietary exclusion of Phe.

Stigmata: *ABCDEFGH*

> *A*utistic behaviour
> *B*lue eyes
> *C*erebral palsy (visual perception and visual motor skills – more than a third never learn to talk or walk)
> o*D*our (characteristically mousy)
> *E*czema
> *F*its
> *G*rowth is diminished
> *H*air fair (pigmentation deficient)

Tay–Sachs disease (cerebromacular degeneration; amaurotic family idiocy) Autosomal recessive in children.

Defect of Hexosaminidase A – leads to gradual accumulation of *g*angliosode *G*M2 in *G*rey matter.

Commonest in *A*shkenazi Jews.

Earliest sign is hyper-*A*cusis (exaggerated startle).

> T'*AY*'–Sachs: hexosaminidase-*A*

Noted sign is macular cherry red spot.

Hurler's disease (gargoylism) Accumulation of mucopolysaccharidoses in tissues including brain.

Stigmata: *THICK*

> *THICK* long bones
> *H*epatosplenomegaly
> *I*ncrease in head size (disproportionately large)
> *C*orneal clouding
> *K*yphosis

X-linked recessive disorders

Lesch–Nyan syndrome Deficiency of hypoxanthine phosphoribosyl transferase (HGPRT) in purine metabolism.

Features: Le*SCH*

*H*yperuricaemia
*C*horeoathetosis
*S*eizures, *S*pasticity, *S*elf-mutilation, *S*mall skull

Fragile X syndrome (Martin–Bell–Renpenning syndrome)
Occurs in 1:1000 of general male population.

Second most common known cause of mental retardation in males.

Fragile site [Xq27] – revealed by fragility test (lymphocyte culture in folate deficient medium).

Stigmata in males:
  – perseverative speech which is high pitched and often nasal
  – associated with:
      attention-deficit disorder and autistic disorder (20% of autistics have fragile X syndrome)
      variable degree of mental retardation
      short stature
      flexible joints
      large   ears (floppy)
              chin (prognathism)
              testicles (macro-orchidism).

Females (1:2000) usually carriers but can express phenotypical features and have mental retardation.

Conditions featuring trinucleatide repeat:

Fragile X – CGG
Huntington's disease – CAG
Myotonic dystrophy – CTG

X-linked dominant disorder
Rett's disorder Progressive degenerative disorder affecting solely females.

Development is normal for first six months of life.

Then manifest:

*H*and *S*tereotypies (loss of purposeful movements)	*S*eizures (75%)
*H*and wringing	*S*coliosis
*H*ead growth halts or slows down	*S*pasticity
	*S*mall feet
*H*aphazard movements gait and trunk (ataxia)	*S*peech deficits (receptive/expressive language)
*H*yperventilation	*S*ocial interaction/engagement is lost

Multifactorial disorders

Schizophrenia Familial aggregation of schizophrenia has been shown in family, twin and adoption studies.

Lifetime risk of schizophrenia in relatives of schizophrenic proband is shown in Table 13.2:

Table 13.2   Lifetime risk of schizophrenia in relatives

Relation	Lifetime risk (%)
Parent	6
Sibling	10
Sibling (a parent is also affected)	17
Children	13
Children (both parents affected)	46
Grandchildren	4
Uncles, aunts, nephews, nieces	3
Unrelated	1

Modes of inheritance **Single major locus** (no such locus has been found), **polygenic** and **multifactorial**. **Mixed model** is also proposed with major gene operating against multifactorial background.

Linkage studies: implicated several genes. None replicated or sufficiently supported. (5q; 11q; 6p-HLA9).

Association with velocardiofacial syndrome (CATCH22) involving chromosome C22q.

Affective disorders **Family studies:** first degree relatives of unipolar depressives have an increased risk of only unipolar depression. First degree relatives of bipolar patients have an increased risk of both unipolar and bipolar illness.

Twin studies: monozygotic : dizygotic concordance ratio is approximately 2:1 for unipolar disorder and 4:1 for bipolar disorder.

Adoption studies:
- 26% of biological parents of bipolar patients have mood disorder
- 28% of biological parents of bipolar adoptees have mood disorder
- 12% of adoptive parents of bipolar adoptees have mood disorder.

Linkage studies: some familial links of bipolar illness to glucose-6-phosphate deficiency and colour blindness (Xp).

Also in some pedigrees linkage to chromosome 11. However, results lack replication.

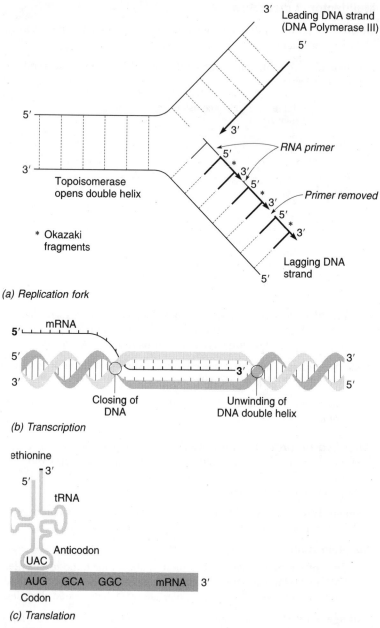

(a) Replication fork

(b) Transcription

(c) Translation

Figure 13.1

Alcoholism Family studies: runs in families. Relatives of alcoholics more likely to be alcoholics.

Twin studies: concordance in monozygotic twins higher than that for dizygotic twins.

Adoption studies: parental alcoholism increases risk of alcoholism in males (x4).

Others There is a significant genetic contribution to the familial aggregation of:

– phobia
– social phobia (risk to relatives $\times 3$)
– panic disorder (risk to relatives $\times 10$)
– obsessive–compulsive disorder
– eating disorders.

14 Neuroimaging

Neuroimaging is divided into structural and functional. Some techniques provide both types of information.

Structural neuroimaging

Skull radiography

Using X-rays, the bones of the skull can be visualized. It is useful in detecting bone pathology and trauma. Largely superseded by CT. Often used in accident and emergency departments as a screening measure following head injury.

Computerized tomography (CT)

Like skull radiography, CT images are dependent upon the attenuation, i.e. the loss of energy and slowing, of X-ray photons as they pass through tissues of varying density. Having passed through tissue the emerging X-ray beams are detected and recorded using scintillation counters and from this data, computer images are mathematically reconstructed and displayed as radiodensity maps. High-density matter, such as bone, appears white and low-density matter, e.g. cerebrospinal fluid, appears black. The CT scan image can be enhanced with the aid of contrast media.

Magnetic resonance imaging (MRI)

The application of a strong magnetic field aligns the atomic spin axes and produces precession (axial rotation specific to each atom). The delivery of a radiofrequency impulse imparting energy promotes a shift of some nuclei to a higher quantum level (resonance). Subsequent return to their previous level (relaxation) results in the emission of radiofrequency waves which are detected as the magnetic resonance signal. Tissue relaxation is described as T-1 (longitudinal plane – one) and T-2 (transverse plane – two). Alteration of the radiofrequency impulses allows T-1/T-2 weighting permitting modulation of image specificity. This then allows the derivation of functional information in addition to high resolution structural data.

Functional neuroimaging

Single photon emission computed tomography (SPECT/SPET)

A ligand or compound labelled radioactively with an isotope that emits γ photons (radiolabelled ligand/radioisotope) is administered by inhalation, ingestion or intravenous injection. The ligand or compound is chosen on the basis of its specificity for receptors or chemical processes. Its activity can be monitored by computer analysis of its γ photon emissions. From this data images can be constructed called SPECT/SPET scans. Various ligands are used to study receptor density and several compounds are used to examine regional cerebral blood flow (rCBF).

Positron emission tomography (PET)

PET relies on very short-acting radioactive isotopes (e.g. F^{18}, N^{13}, C^{11}) which require on-site synthesis in a **cyclotron**. The positrons that these isotopes emit collide with electrons to produce two gamma photons travelling in diametrically opposite directions. These are then detected and recorded providing data for computer processing from which an image (PET scan) is constructed. PET is more expensive than SPECT but provides images of much greater resolution.

Functional MRI (fMRI)

MRI manipulation can be used to derive functional information (see above). fMRI uses the non-invasive blood oxygenation level dependent (BOLD) technique to map cortical activation.

Magnetic encephalography (MEG)

MEG is a non-invasive technique that characterizes per millisecond brain electrophysiology by analysing cerebral biomagnetic fields. It can be combined with structural MRI and is useful for:

- localizing epileptiform activity
- mapping of sensorimotor cortex prior to neurosurgery
- characterizing spontaneous abnormal rhythms associated with various neuropathologies.

Magnetic resonance spectroscopy (MRS)

In principle, MRS is similar to structural MRI; however, its focus on chemical composition enables the detection of blood flow and metabolic changes.

Significant psychiatric neuroimaging findings
(For summary see Appendix)

Schizophrenia

- Structural: CT and MRI
  - Non-progressive lateral and third ventricular enlargement.
  - Reduction in size of superior temporal gyrus, medial temporal lobe and frontal lobe.
  - Structural abnormalities have been noted in several regions of the brain: hippocampus, parahippocampal gyrus, amygdala and planum temporale.
  - Increased ventricular size, especially lateral.
- Functional: PET; SECT; fMRI; MRS and MEG
  - Hypofrontality (NB some studies have shown ↑ rCBF to L hemisphere and L globus pallidus)
  - Liddle's symptom clusters
    psychomotor poverty; ↓ rCBF in L and medial prefrontal cortex
    disorganization; ↓ rCBF in Broca's area and ↑ perfusion of R medial prefrontal cortex
    reality distortion; ↑ rCBF in left hippocampal formation
    ↑ response to sensory stimulation
    ↓ response of frontal cortex while performing cognitive tasks
    ↓ synthesis ↑ turnover of dorsolateral prefrontal cortex membrane phospholipids.

Affective disorders

- Structural
  - ↓ Volume of frontal cortex, brainstem, caudate and vermis.
  - ↑ Ventricular size (inconsistent) ? related to cognitive changes and atrophy.
  - Deep white matter hyperintensities in elderly depressives and possibly those with bipolar disorder (associated with poor response to treatment).
  - Hippocampal atrophy.
  - Pituitary hypertrophy.
  - Adrenal gland hypertrophy.

- Functional
  - Reversible hypofrontality.
  - ↓ Cingulate cortex rCBF in depressed state. Normalizes with clinical recovery.

Anxiety disorders

- Structural
  - ↓ Size of R hippocampus in PTSD.
- Functional
  - ↓ rCBF R parahippocampus in panic disorder.
  - ↓ Benzodiazepine receptor density in several brain regions of anxious patients.

Obsessive–compulsive disorder (OCD)

- Structural
  - ↓ and ↑ of caudate nucleus volume have been noted.
- Functional
  - Caudate nucleus and orbitofrontal cortex changes in metabolism and rCBF.
  - rCBF changes normalize with clinical improvement.

Dementia

- Structural
  - Marked progressive ventricular enlargement is noted in Alzheimer's disease.
  - The degree of generalized cortical atrophy and pattern of localized atrophy varies according to aetiology.
- Functional
  - ↓ rCBF, particularly in temporal regions.
  - ↑ Phosphomonoesterases in Alzheimer's disease.

Alcoholism

- Structural
  - Cerebral and cerebellar cortical atrophy.
  - Extent of cortical atrophy correlates with degree of cognitive impairment.
- Functional
  - ↓ rCBF (non-specific) correlates with severity of alcohol abuse.

15 *Peptidergic neurotransmission and neuroendocrinology*

Peptidergic neurotransmission

Peptides consist of two or more amino acids joined by **peptide bonds**. They are smaller than proteins with a molecular weight less than 10 kDaltons. Their structure is described left to right from the N-terminus (end with an amino group) to the C-terminus (end with carboxyl group). Neuropeptides are synthesized as prepropeptides. These possess an N-terminus signal sequence consisting of hydrophobic amino acids. The signal sequence ('pre' portion of prepropeptide) facilitates entry of the prepropeptide into endoplasmic reticulum where it is cleaved to form a propeptide. This is then chemically modified prior to secretion.

Catabolism of peptides is carried out by specific peptidases that are important in terminating their neurotransmitter functions.

Neuropeptides (peptide transmitters) differ from classic transmitters in several important ways (see Table 15.1).

Co-localization (coexistence) of transmitters

Sir John Eccles formalized Dale's principle stating that the different terminals of a particular neurone/cell should behave in a similar fashion

Table 15.1 Classic and peptide neurotransmitters

	Classic neurotransmitter	Peptide neurotransmitter
Precursor synthesis	No	Yes (pre-pro-peptide)
Converting enzymes	No	Yes
Synthesized in soma	No (not usually)	Yes
Synthesized in terminals	Yes	No (not usually)
Effective concentrations	Micromolar/nanomolar	Picomolar
Relative rate of synthesis	Fast	Slow
Receptor affinity	High	Low
Receptor potency	Low	High
Neuronal re-uptake	Yes	No (not significant)

and thereby release the same transmitter. The assertion is that neurones display chemical unity/uniformity and the principle does not address the number of transmitters a neurone/cell uses.

Transmitter co-localization is a relatively recent discovery which adds to the complexity of neurotransmission. Co-localized transmitters may act as **neuromodulators**. That is, they modulate the action of a coexistent transmitter rather than effecting actions themselves. This may be achieved by interacting with the transmitter directly or through receptors on the same or different neurones.

Table 15.2 gives examples that have been shown to coexist.

Table 15.2 Neurotransmitter co-localization

Neurotransmitter	Co-localized neuropeptide	Neurones
Acetylcholine	Vasoactive intestinal peptide	Cortical and parasympathetic
Dopamine	Cholecystokinin	Ventrotegmental
Noradrenaline	Neuropeptide Y	Brainstem
GABA	Somatostatin	Hippocampal
Serotonin	TRH and Substance P	Medulla

Classification

Neuropeptides can be grouped as follows:

1 Hypothalamic releasing hormones
  – corticotrophin-releasing hormone (CRH)
  – thyrotrophin-releasing hormone (TRH)
  – somatostatin
  – gonadotrophin-releasing hormone
  – growth hormone-releasing hormone (GHRH).
2 Pituitary hormones
  – oxytocin ⎤
  – vasopressin ⎦ (posterior pituitary)
  – adrenocorticotrophic hormone (ACTH) ⎫ from basophils
  – thyroid stimulating hormone (TSH) ⎭
  – luteinizing hormone (LH)
  – follicle-stimulating hormone (FSH)
  – growth hormone (GH) ⎤ from acidophils
  – prolactin (PRL). ⎦
3 Gut-brain peptides
  – vasoactive intestinal peptide (VIP)
  – cholecystokinin (CCK)
  – Substance P
  – neuropeptide Y

- neurotensin
- insulin
- glucagon.
4 Opioid peptides
  - leu-enkephalin
  - met-enkephalin
  - β-endorphin
  - dynorphin.
5 Others
  - calcitonin-gene-related peptide (CGRP)
  - bradykinin.

Endogenous opioid peptides

These fall into three groups derived from separate precursor polypeptides:

Enkephalins Derived from proenkephalins. Are widely distributed throughout central and peripheral nervous systems. Met-enkephalin and leu-enkephalin are pentapeptides.

Endorphins Derived from proopiomelanocortin (POMC) in pituitary anterior and intermediate lobes and hypothalamic arcuate nucleus. POMC gives rise to β-endorphin and also contains amino acid sequences for β-lipotropin, ACTH and melanocyte-stimulating hormone.

Dynorphins Derived from prodynorphin.

There are three main classes of central nervous system opioid receptors: μ (mu), κ (kappa) and δ (delta). These are concentrated in hypothalamic, limbic and sensory brain regions and in particular the amygdala and periaqueductal grey matter.

The G-protein coupled opioid receptors inhibit neurotransmission by diminishing the release of other neurotransmitters (DA, ACh, 5-HT).

κ receptors are calcium-channel linked (decrease Ca^{2+} entry), as may be μ and δ receptors in certain tissues.

μ receptors and δ receptors are also potassium-channel linked (increase K^+ conductance) and all three types of receptor can inhibit adenylate cyclase.

Endogenous opioids are involved in addiction, dependence, analgesia, learning and memory, and opioid receptor changes have been implicated in affective disorders and schizophrenia.

Vasoactive intestinal peptide (VIP)

Found in autonomic ganglia, intestinal and respiratory tracts and in the cerebral cortex, hypothalamus, amygdala and hippocampus. VIP stimulates the release of ACTH, growth hormone and prolactin and inhibits the release of somatostatin. It also produces neuronal excitation.

Somatostatin

Plays an important role in inhibiting the release of growth hormone and generally has inhibitory effects. It is concentrated in the cerebral cortex and limbic system and is diminished in dementia (Alzheimer's). It has an excitatory effect on hippocampal pyramidal cells.

Cholecystokinin (CCK)

CCK-8 is the most prevalent of its three forms (CCK-33 and CCK-39) and is found especially in the amygdala, hippocampus and cerebral cortex, where it has excitatory effects. It is thought to act on dopamine pathways and is important in mechanisms of satiety, analgesia, panic and anxiety.

Neuroendocrinology

Specialized hypothalamic cells release neuropeptides that act on anterior pituitary cells to release peptide hormones. These then enter the systemic circulation and are able to act on specific organs/tissues (Figures 15.1 and 15.2).

There are several neuroendocrine axes that function in this manner: they are usually described with particular reference to the end-organ, e.g. the adrenal and thyroid axes or the specific hormone of interest, e.g. the growth hormone and the gonadotrophin axes.

These neuropeptides and the end-organ hormones exert negative-feedback control. The release of the hypothalamic neuropeptides is also influenced by neurotransmitters.

Neuroendocrine studies have revealed significant changes in several psychiatric disorders.

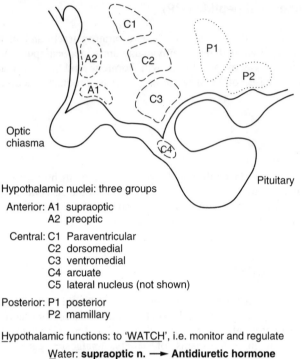

Optic
chiasma

Pituitary

Hypothalamic nuclei: three groups

Anterior: A1 supraoptic
         A2 preoptic

Central: C1 Paraventricular
         C2 dorsomedial
         C3 ventromedial
         C4 arcuate
         C5 lateral nucleus (not shown)

Posterior: P1 posterior
           P2 mamillary

Hypothalamic functions: to 'WATCH', i.e. monitor and regulate

      Water: **supraoptic n. → Antidiuretic hormone**
      Appetite: **ventromedial n. (satiety centre); lateral n. (hunger centre)**
      Temperature: **cells in preoptic n. sensitive to blood temperature**
      Cardiovascular system: **preoptic area ↓Heart rate**
                                    posterior area ↑Heart rate

Figure 15.1 *Hypothalamic nuclei*

HPA-axis

Corticotrophin releasing hormone (CRH) from the hypothalamic paraventricular nucleus (PVN) travels in the hypothalamic-hypophyseal-
portal-system to the anterior pituitary where it acts to yield adrenocorticotrophic hormone (ACTH) from proopiomelanocortin (POMC). ACTH
released into the bloodstream acts on the adrenal cortex resulting in the
release of cortisol (see Figure 15.3).

The brain possess two types of 'steroid receptor':

- **mineralocorticoid receptors (type I)** have a high affinity for cortisol
  and are to be found mainly in the septo-hippocampal complex.
- **glucocorticoid receptors (type II)** have less affinity for cortisol and
  are more widely distributed.

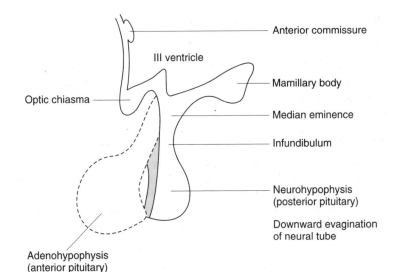

Figure 15.2   *Pituitary gland*

Both types of receptor participate in HPA-axis negative feedback. Negative feedback has been shown to be fast, intermediate and slow. Slow feedback occurs over a period of hours and involves the inhibition of pituitary ACTH synthesis. Intermediate feedback occurs over a period of minutes. It is concentration-dependent and diminishes ACTH secretion. Fast feedback is rate-sensitive and inhibits ACTH secretion in a matter of seconds following a rapid increase of plasma cortisol.

Normally the HPA-axis has a circadian rhythm. Peak cortisol secretion occurs early morning and it falls to its lowest late evening.

HPA abnormalities

Depression

- Cortisol hypersecretion (50% of patients) with increased urinary excretion (2 × normal).
- Adrenal gland volume shows 70% ↑ (MRI).
- Pituitary gland enlargement.
- ↑ CSF CRH (depressed patients and suicides).
- ↓ CRH receptor binding sites in frontal cortex of suicides.
- Dexamethasone suppression test non-suppression (50–70% of major depressives; >90% of those with psychotic depression).*

- Blunted ACTH/cortisol responses to CRH.
- Blunted ACTH/cortisol responses to ipsapirone (5-HT$_{1A}$ agonist).
- HPA abnormalities (particularly hypercortisolaemia and DST non-suppression) usually normalize with clinical recovery.

* Not specific, also found in: OCD; dementia; panic disorder; eating disorders; alcohol withdrawal; normal population (5–10%).

Schizophrenia

- Normal ACTH/cortisol response to CRH.
- Dexamethasone non-suppression may occur in acute episodes of schizophrenia (contentious findings), however, it has rarely been observed in patients with chronic schizophrenia.

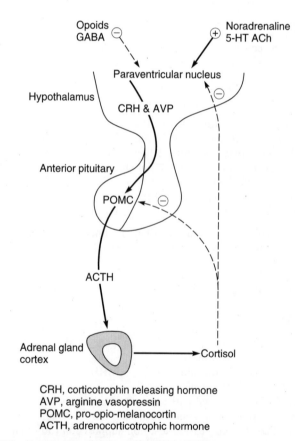

CRH, corticotrophin releasing hormone
AVP, arginine vasopressin
POMC, pro-opio-melanocortin
ACTH, adrenocorticotrophic hormone

Figure 15.3 *Hypothalmic-pituitary-adrenal axis (HPA)*

Alzheimer's disease

- Hypercortisolaemia.
- Dexamethasone non-suppression (>50% of patients).

Thyroid axis abnormalities Hypothalamic thyrotropin releasing hormone (TRH) travels in the hypophyseal portal system to the anterior pituitary gland where it stimulates the synthesis and release of thyroid stimulating hormone (TSH). TSH releases the thyroid hormones triiodothyronine (T_3) and thyroxine (T_4) from the thyroid gland. Axis function is influenced by TSH and thyroid hormone negative feedback and is inhibited by somatostatin.

Depression

- ↑ TSH levels (subclinical hypothyroidism) especially common in those with BAD.
- Blunted response to TRH stimulation in about 30% of depressives; this remains despite clinical recovery in about 15% and seems to be associated with increased likelihood of relapse.
- ↑ CSF TRH levels
- 20% have anti-thyroid antibodies (more than twice the level in normal population).

Prolactin axis abnormalities

Prolactin (PRL) is released from anterior pituitary cells in response to thyrotropin releasing hormone (TRH), arginine-vasopressin (AVP) and vasoactive-intestinal peptide (VIP). Dopamine inhibits the release of PRL whereas serotonin and its amino-acid precursor tryptophan enhance its release (indirectly).

Depression PRL release is blunted in response to:

- tryptophan
- d-fenfluramine (causes 5-HT release and inhibits its re-uptake)
- clomipramine.

Growth hormone axis abnormalities

Pituitary growth hormone (GH) release is stimulated by GH-releasing hormone (GHRH) and inhibited by somatostatin. The release of these neuropeptides is influenced by neurotransmitters ACh, DA and NA (Figure 15.4).

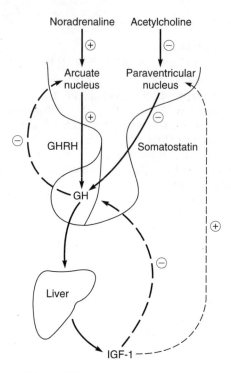

GH, growth hormone
GHRH, growth hormone releasing hormone
IGF-1, insulin-like growth factor

Figure 15.4 *Growth hormone axis*

GH is released in pulses and peaks with the onset of slow-wave sleep. Its release is stimulated by stress, hypoglycaemia, exercise, sleep, surgery and pyrexia and inhibited by negative feedback.

Depression

- GH release is blunted in response to:
  - hypoglycaemia (insulin tolerance test)
  - **clonidine** (α_2-agonist)
  - **desipramine**.
- GH release increased in response to **pyridostigmine** (anticholinesterase).
- Reduced nocturnal secretion.
- ↓ CSF somatostatin.

Schizophrenia and Alzheimer's disease (tentative finding)

- $\downarrow$ CSF somatostatin.

Neuroendocrine abnormalities in eating disorders and OCD

Anorexia nervosa

- $\downarrow$ plasma T_3 (NB T_4 level normal).
- $\downarrow$ plasma oestrogen and gonadotrophins.

Anorexia nervosa and bulimia nervosa

- $\uparrow$ plasma GH.
- $\uparrow$ plasma cortisol.
- $\uparrow$ plasma CCK.
- Dexamethasone non-suppression.

Obsessive–compulsive disorder (OCD)

- Blunted prolactin and cortisol responses to **d-fenfluramine** challenge.
- Normal responses to **clonidine** and **desipramine** challenge.
- Normal dexamethasone suppression.
- Enhanced GH response to **pyridostigmine.**

16 *Statistics and epidemiology*

Statistics

Statistics is the mathematics of data collection, description and interpretation.

Terms used in statistics **Variable**: a characteristic that can be experimentally measured or quantified.

Described as **independent** when controlled and manipulated by the experimenter and **dependent** when describing the attributes influenced by independent variables. Dependent variables are usually measures of outcome or effect.

Variables can also be described as **qualitative** or **quantitative.**

Quantitative data is that which can be described and categorized numerically. Qualitative data is that which cannot. Consequently qualitative data can only be measured using nominal or ordinal scales whereas quantitative data can also be measured using interval and ratio scales. These are described in Chapter 4.

Quantitative variables are either **discrete** or **continuous**. The latter can have any value of a specific measure whereas discrete variables are categorical and fixed.

Statistics is divided into descriptive and inferential:

Descriptive statistics

Summarize and organize data.

Frequency distributions

Values are arranged according to frequency. Can be presented in a **table** as individual values or **cumulative frequency**.

- discrete probability distributions; **binomial** distribution and **Poisson** distribution.
- continuous probability distributions; **normal** distribution and χ^2 (chi-square) distribution.

Data can be presented graphically in a variety of ways: **scatter diagram, bar-graph, frequency polygon, cumulative plot** and **histogram.**

Summary statistics

Describe central tendency and extent of dispersion or degree of variability.

Measures of central tendency: mean, median and mode The **mean** (average) is the sum of the values divided by their number. It considers all the values and its use is restricted to interval and ratio variables. It is sensitive to extreme values (skewed distributions).

The **median** (50th percentile) is the middle value when they are ranked in order and it divides the distribution into two equally sized groups. (NB Applies to odd number of values. With even number of values, the median is calculated as the mean of the two middle values.) The median is less sensitive to extreme values than the mean and can also be used for values measured on an ordinal scale.

The **mode** is the most common value within a distribution, i.e. that occurring most frequently. It can be used for data measured on a nominal scale (see Table 16.1).

Table 16.1 Measurement scales to which measures of central tendency can be applied

Measure	Scale			
	nominal	ordinal	interval	ratio
mean			+	+
median		+	+	+
mode	+	+	+	+

Measures of dispersion: range, variance, standard deviation and standard error The **range** is the difference between the highest and lowest values. It is distorted by extreme values and can be applied only to values measured on an interval or ratio scale.

The **variance** uses all the values in the distribution calculating their deviation from the mean. The differences between the mean and each value are squared and then summed. The result is then divided by the sample size minus 1. Sample and population variances denoted by s^2 and σ^2

$s^2 = [\Sigma (x - x)^2]/n - 1$ for sample size n with mean x.

$\sigma^2 = [\Sigma (x - \mu)^2]/N$ population size N with mean μ.

High variance reflects a wide dispersion of data values. The closer the values are to the mean the smaller the variance. Note that the units used to express variance are the square of those of the data.

The **standard deviation** (σ) is the square root of the variance and is expressed in the same units as the data. In a normal distribution 95% of the values lie within two standard deviations of the mean. Normal distribution values can be standardized by transforming them to a **z score** (standard normal variate, Z). This denotes the distance from the mean in terms of standard deviations and is calculated by subtracting the mean from the original value and dividing the result by the standard deviation. The sign (+ or –) of the z score denotes whether it is above or below the mean.

$$Z = (x - \mu)/\sigma$$

The **standard error of the mean (s.e.m.)** measures the extent of variation of the sample means and provides an approximation of the true population value. It is calculated by dividing the standard deviation by the square root of the sample size ($\sigma/\sqrt{n}$).

Inferential statistics

This involves making inferences about population characterisitcs based on sample data. The statistics are based on probability theory and the tests are described as **parametric** and **non-parametric.**

Hypothesis testing

When comparing groups with respect to a particular variable, hypotheses are posed that involve true population differences. A **one-tailed** test is used if differences are hypothesized to occur in only one direction, otherwise a **two-tailed** test is used.

First the **null hypothesis** is specified, H_0, that there is no difference between the groups. If then statistically it can be shown that any observed differences between the groups are unlikely to be due to chance alone then the null hypothesis can be rejected in favour of the **alternative hypothesis, H_1**; that there is a difference between the groups. The likelihood or the extent to which it is probable that the difference occurred by chance alone is expressed in terms of significance at a specified level.

Misinterpretation of results can lead to two types of error:

   – **type I error**; incorrectly rejecting the null hypothesis (wrongly concluding that there are group differences). The probability of committing a type I error is denoted by α and represents the **significance level**.

– **type II error**; incorrectly rejecting the alternate hypothesis (wrongly concluding that there are no group differences). The probability of committing a type II error is denoted by β.

The **power of a test** is the probability that the null hypothesis will be correctly rejected, i.e. it is false and recognized as such. This is equal to $1 - \beta$.

p value is the probability of obtaining an outcome through chance alone. However, it conveys no information about the size or direction of any difference.

Confidence intervals: the specified level of confidence denotes the likelihood that the population mean lies within the stated interval, i.e. it indicates the degree of certainty that can be applied to the accuracy of the population estimate.

Tests **Parametric tests**: at least one of the variables is measured on an interval or ratio scale.

– *t*-**test**: compares the means of two samples to determine the likelihood of any difference occurring by chance. It consists of an independent variable (nominal or categorical) and a dependent variable (quantitative or continuous). A t-test can be **paired** (sample means are from matched groups or the same group) or **unpaired** (samples are independent).

– **ANOVA (analysis of variance)**: compares the means of many groups. Described as **one-way** when there is only one independent variable and **two-way** when there are two. It involves calculating the **F ratio,** which is the degree of variation between groups relative to the variation within groups.

– **Correlation:** the extent to which two variables are related. Correlation can be **positive** or **negative** or the variables may be uncorrelated. Correlation is given a value -1.00 to $+1.00$ depending on the strength of the correlation and its direction. This is called Pearson's correlation coefficient.

– **Regression analysis:** describes the association between several predictor variables and an outcome variable.

Non-parametric tests These are used when both the dependent and independent variables are nominal or ordinal.

– **Chi-square test (χ^2)** ; makes comparisons using a contingency table in which the rows and columns represent the different variables. Chi-square is the ratio of observed to expected frequencies in

contingency table cells and indicates whether there is a significant difference from that which would be expected if no association was present. If the expected cell frequencies are small than a **Fisher exact test** is used instead.
- **Mann–Whitney U test:** this is the non-parametric equivalent of the independent samples t-test and is used for ranked ordinal data.
- **Correlation**: this can be tested using a variety of tests resulting in the correlation coefficients: Spearman's (ρ), Cohen's (κ), Kendall's (τ).

Epidemiology

This is the study of the distribution and determinants of disease in a population. It is a structure for describing diseases.

Uses of clinical epidemiology

- aetiology
- natural and clinical history
- intervention

- risk of onset
- prognosis
- evidenced based practice
- risk of recurrence.

Basic Description

Measurement of disease

Prevalence The number of cases in a population at one point in time.

Prevalence rate (PR) The number of cases in a population at one point in time/number of people at risk

Specify: Point PR (data collected at one time), Period PR (data collected over a defined period).

Incidence The number of new cases arising over a given period.

Incidence rate The number of new cases arising over a given period/ number of people at risk OR sum of length of time at risk.

Cumulative incidence rate The number of new cases over a given period/number of people disease free in at risk population.

Prevalence rate (approximates to) → incidence rate × average disease duration.

Comparing disease

Relative risk Risk of disease in exposed/risk of disease in unexposed.

In plain English: *How many more times do exposed persons become diseased than non-exposed?*

Attributable risk (risk difference) Difference in rate of occurrence (incidence) between exposed and non-exposed.

In plain English: *How many new cases are due to the risk factor?*

Attributable fraction Attributable risk/total rate of occurrence in exposed population.

In plain English: *What proportion of disease is due to the risk factor?*

Population attributable risk The excess risk of disease in a population multiplied by the prevalence of exposure.

In plain English: *How many cases in the population are due to the risk factor?*

Causation

Causation or aetiology refers to the determinants of disease onset.

A risk factor is something positively associated with disease onset but not sufficient to cause the disease.

Cause

Predisposing factors   Create a susceptibility
Precipitating factors   Closely associated with disease expression

Onset

Pathophysiological factors   Mechanism by which a disease is expressed
Pathoplastic factors   Influence the expression of disease

Course

Perpetuating factors   Maintains an established disease
Prognostic factors   Influence a disease outcome

Establishing a cause This is an important part of every day practice. Many unifactoral disorders have an identified cause based on Koch's postulates (1882):

- the organism must be present in every case of the disease.
- the organism must be isolated and grown.
- the organism must be able to cause the disease when inoculated into susceptible host.
- the organism must be recovered from that host and identified.

When such experimental evidence is not available or complex multifactoral systems are involved, Austin Bradford Hill's criteria may be used (1965).

- Temporality – the cause precedes the effect.
- Strength – exposure vs non-exposure produces large difference in disease.
- Dose-response – increased exposure produced increased effect.
- Reversibility – reduction in exposure reduces disease occurrence.
- Consistency – similar association has been replicated.
- Specificity – one cause leads to one effect.
- Plausibility – the association is concordant with current knowledge.

Table 16.2   Evidence of cause from Studies

Study design	Additional evidence	Strength of hypothesis
Hypothesis alone	Plausibility	
Case report	Specificity	
Meta-analysis	Consistency	
Cross-sectional	Dose-response	
Case-control	Strength	
Cohort study	Temporality	
Clinical trial	Reversibility	Strongest

There is no 'gold-standard' for deciding whether an association is causal. Causal inference is the process whereby the decision is reached. In assessing an association arising from a study, first ask could the observed association be due to:

- bias in selection or measurement?
- confounding factors?
- chance?

If not, then the null hypothesis of no difference can be rejected and a causal explanation for the association sought.

Diagnosis

Diagnosis is the process by which diseases are identified. When performed on a large scale the term screening is used.

An ideal diagnostic test should be:

*S*ensitive
*S*pecific
*S*imple
*S*afe
*S*ound (i.e. reliable!)

The relationship between a theoretical test and disease is illustrated in the Diagnostic matrix.

Table 16.3 Diagnostic matrix (analysis of a test)

	Disease present Reject null hypothesis	*Disease absent* Accept null hypothesis
Positive test	a	b
Negative test	c	d
Sensitivity	a/a + c	
Specificity	d/b + d	
Positive predictive value	a/a + b	
Negative predictive value	d/c + d	
Efficiency	a + d/a + b + c + d	

In plain English:

Sensitivity   *The proportion of people with the disease who have a positive test.*

Specificity	The proportion of people without the disease who have a negative test.
Positive PV	Proportion of people who have the disease in those who tested positive.
Negative PV	Proportion of people not having the disease in those with a negative test.
Efficiency or Accuracy	Proportion of all tests that are correct.

For serious diseases, it is appropriate to have less stringent criteria (or cut-off point), thus increasing sensitivity but reducing specificity by introducing false positives.

For diseases suspected on other criteria, it is appropriate to have stringent criteria (or cut-off point) thus increased specificity at the expense of sensitivity or false negatives.

What are odds and odds ratios?

Odds There is some confusion over these terms and their application to assessing the accuracy of a test. Odds is **NOT** identical to probability or relative risk, but in fact is a ratio of probabilities expressed as:

$$\text{Odds} = \frac{\text{Probability of an event}}{1 - \text{Probability of an event}}$$

Odds ratio The odds ratio or likelihood ratio is the probability of a test result in those with the disease divided by the probability of the result in those without the disease.

$$\text{Odds ratio} = \frac{\text{Sensitivity}}{1 - \text{Specificity}}$$

Prognosis and Treatment

Prognosis is the prediction of the future course of a disease. Prognostic factors are thus variables which influence disease course, once it is established.

| Natural history | – Is the course of the disease without intervention. |
| Clinical course | – Is the course of the disease with medical intervention. |

Measures of outcome

Symptoms and signs – severity, response, remission, relapse
Markers   – Diagnostic tests, social function, handicap
Diagnosis   – recovery, recurrence
Mortality   – survival

Survival analysis

The time-to-death from the point of recruitment (zero-time) is collected. This can be plotted in a survival curve indicating the cumulative probability of surviving each time interval preceding the point of data entry. Patients lost from a study are removed or **censored**.

Bias in prognostic studies

Sampling bias Refers to an effect of outcome based on characteristics of patients determined by the recruitment process.

Assembly bias Patients differ at baseline in factors (which influence outcome) other than that under study.

Migration bias Once under way patients from one cohort leave or swap non-randomly.

Measurement bias Patients from one cohort have differing detection of the outcome than a comparison cohort.

Controlling for bias

Randomization Assigning patients to groups randomly gives an equal chance of known and unknown factors to be distributed equally.

Restriction Excluding patients with potentially confounding variables.

Matching Patients under study compared with patients with the same characteristics except for those under study.

Stratification At the analysis stage, subgroups with same characteristics selected.

Inception cohort Patients are recruited at a similarly early stage in their disease (without this technique the study becomes a **survival cohort**).

Treatment studies

Clinical trials are a special form of cohort study, in which one factor (treatment) but no other, varies between two groups (experimental and control).

Uncontrolled trials Compare the condition before and after treatment in a single patient group.

Controlled trials Utilize a comparison arm such as placebo, second drug or usual treatment.

Randomization The process whereby patients are allocated to either arm without bias.

Blinding Participants and researchers do not know the allocation of treatment arms (double-blind).

NB: blinding at the stage of allocation and analysis can also occur.

Problems in treatment studies

Generalizability The study may show the treatment works under ideal study conditions (i.e. it demonstrates efficacy) but does the treatment work in ordinary circumstances (effectiveness)?

Hawthorne effect Participants change their behaviour because they are being studied.

Halo effect Researchers put results into prejudged categories.

Compliance If participants are included in analysis regardless of their participation after treatment begins this is **intention-to-treat** analysis. If only participants who completed the study are considered, this is **completor analysis**.

Regression to the mean If patients with extreme results are recruited, results are likely to improve for statistical reasons (see also Chapter 4 Psychological assessment).

Types of study

Table 16.4

Type of Study	Subtypes
Observational studies	
Descriptive	
Analytic	Ecological (correlational)
	Cross-sectional (prevalence)
	Case-control
	Cohort (follow-up)
Interventional studies	
Clinical trials	Randomized
	Non-randomized
Community trials	

Special types of study

Case-control studies Patients with the disease are compared to those without. All other factors should be equal. Inquiry is made retrospectively for past risks (exposure). Data on exposure factors may be collected before or after the development of the disease.

Advantages:	measures rare diseases, studies multiple risk factors, deals with long latency.
Problems:	selection bias, recall bias, confounding factors.

Cohort studies

People free of disease are stratified into those with and without the putative
  risk factor and are followed longitudinally when the development of
  disease is noted.

Advantages: measures rare causes, and incidence, demonstrates
                  temporal pattern.
Problems: drops-outs, cost, time.

Appendices

Appendix 1

Theorists in the analytic psychiatry, social sciences and psychology

Author	Key association	Author	Key association
Abraham	Psychoanalyst	Kohut	Self-psychology
Adler	Individual psychology	Kretschmer	Body-build
Allport	Humanistic psychology	Kubler-Ross	Death and dying
Bannister	Repertory grid	Latance	Social impact theory
Bateson	Double-bind	Lidz	Marital skew
Berne	Transactional analysis	Lorenz	Imprinting
Binet	Intellectual ability	Maslow	Hierarchy of needs
Bion	Group therapy	McClelland	Achievement
Borgadus	Social distance scale	Mechanic	Illness behaviour
Bowlby	Loss	Meyer	Psychobiology
Broca	Expressive dysphasia	Milgram	Obedience
Cannon-Bard	Thalamic emotion theory	Mowrer	Drives
		Osgood	Congruity theory
Cattel	Personality trait theory	Parkes	Bereavement
Ellis	Rational-emotive therapy	Parsons	Sick role
		Pavlov	Classical conditioning
Erikson	Psychosocial development	Perls	Gestalt therapy
		Piaget	Cognitive development
Eysenck	Personality theory	Pilowsky	Abnormal illness behaviour
Festinger	Cognitive dissonance theory	Rank	Primal anxiety
Fiedler	Contingency theory	Rogers	Self-theory
Freud, A.	Defence mechanisms	Rogers	Self-concept psychotherpy
Freud, S.	Psychoanalysis		
Fromm-Reichman	Schizophrenogenic mother	Rotter	Locus of control
		Schacter	Cognitive labelling
Goffman	Institutionalization	Seyle	General adaption syndrome
Heider	Balance theory		
Horney	Holistic psychology	Sheldon	Body-types
Hull	Drive-reduction theory	Skinner	Operant conditioning
James-Lange	Causal emotion theory	Sullivan	Interpersonal theory
Jung	Analytical psychology	Thorndike	Law of effect
Kelly	Personal construct theory	Wernicke	Receptive dysphasia
		Winnicott	Object relations
Klein	Object relations	Wolpe	Reciprocal inhibition
Kohlberg	Moral development		

Appendix 2

Theorists psychiatry, psychopathology and diagnosis

Author	Key Association
Asher	Munchausen's syndrome
Bach-y-Ritta	Episodic dyscontrol syndrome
Barker	Hospital addiction syndrome
Beard	Neurasthenia
Bleuler	Schizophrenia
Cameron	Loosening of associations
Ganser	Vorbegehen
Goldstein	Concrete thinking
Gull	Anorexia nervosa
Hare	Pseudohallucination
Kadinsky	Pseudohallucination
Kahn	Anankastic personality
Kasanin	Schizoaffective disorder
Koch	Psychopathic inferiority
Kraepelin	Dementia praecox
Langfeldt	Schizophreniform psychosis
Leonard	Bipolar affective disorder
Meyer-Gross	Oneroid states
Miller	Accident neurosis
Moeli	Vorbeireden
Morgan	Non-fatal deliberate self-harm
Pinel	Manie sans delirie
Prichard	Moral insanity
Russel	Bulimia nervosa
Schneider	Schizophrenic formal thought disorder
Spitz	Anaclitic depression
Stromgen	Brief reactive psychosis

Appendix 3

Summary of antidepressant pharmacology, relative potency of receptor blockade

Drug	5HT/NA Reuptake ratio	Muscarinic blockade	Dopaminergic blockade	$Alpha_1$ blockade	$Alpha_2$ blockade	Histaminic blockade
Adverse effects	Nausea, Anorexia, Insomnia, Anorgasmia	Dry mouth, Blurred vision, Constipation	Extra-pyramidal Hyperprolactinaemia	Hypotension Tachycardia	Priapism	Sedation Weight gain Hypotension
Increasing affinity ←	Citalopram Paroxetine Fluoxetine Trazadone Clomipramine Amitriptyline Imipramine Nortriptyline Desipramine Reboxetine	Amitriptyline Protriptyline Imipramine Clomipramine Nortriptyline Desipramine Fluoxetine Paroxetine Citalopram Trazadone	Nortriptyline Protriptyline Paroxetine Fluoxetine Amitriptyline Imipramine Desipramine Trazadone	Amitriptyline Trazadone Nortriptyline Imipramine Protriptyline Desipramine Bupropion Paroxetine	Nortriptyline Trazadone Amitriptyline Imipramine Bupropion Protriptyline Desipramine Fluoxetine	Amitriptyline Nortriptyline Imipramine Protriptyline Desipramine Trazadone

Appendix 4

Summary of antipsychotic pharmacology, post-synaptic receptor blockade

Drug	D_2	D_1	$5HT_2$	α_1	α_2	H1	M1
Chlorpromazine	✓	✓		✓		**✓**	**✓**
Haloperidol	**✓**			✓		✓	
Thioridazine	✓	✓				✓	**✓**
Clozapine	✓	✓	✓	✓	✓	✓	**✓**
Olanzapine	✓	✓	✓	✓		**✓**	
Risperidone	**✓**	✓	**✓**	**✓**	✓	**✓**	
Sertindole	✓	✓	**✓**	**✓**			
Quetiapine	✓		✓	✓		**✓**	**✓**
Ziprasidone	✓		**✓**	✓		✓	

Bold indicates a strong effect
Atypical antipsychotics show: Limbic selectivity
Reduced D_2 occupancy
Combined D_2 + $5HT_2$ action (risperidone, sertindole, ziprasidone)
Novel non-D_2 action (clozapine, olanzapine, quetiapine)

Appendix 5

Neuroendocrine findings in psychiatric disorders

Test	Depression	Schizophrenia	Eating disorder	Chronic alcohol dependency	OCD	Alzheimer's disease
HPA axis						
DST	Non-suppression (50%)	Suppression (in 90%)	Non-suppression (50%)	Non-suppression (25%)	Normal	Non-suppression (25%)
CRH challenge	Blunted ACTH	Normal	Blunted ACTH	Unknown	Normal	Blunted ACTH
CSF CRH	High (inconsistent)	Normal	High	Unknown	Unknown	Normal
HPT axis						
T3/T4	Normal	Normal	Low	Normal	Normal	Normal
TSH	Normal	Low (15%)	Normal	Normal	Normal	Normal
TRH challenge	Blunted (30%) Augmented (15%)	Normal	Blunted	Unknown	Unknown	Normal
Thyroid autoantibodies	High (20%)	High (10%)	Normal	Unknown	Unknown	Normal
HPG axis						
Oestrogens	Normal	? Low	Low	Normal	Unknown	Unknown
LHRH challenge	Inconsistent	Unknown	Blunted	Unknown	Unknown	Unknown
Prolactin						
Serotonergic challenge	Blunted	Blunted	Unknown	Unknown	Blunted	Unknown
Growth hormone						
Basal	Blunted diurnal rhythm	Inconsistent	High	Normal	Blunted (30%)	Normal
Clonidine challenge	Blunted	Blunted (mild)	Unknown	Unknown	Blunted (30%)	Normal
Insulin challenge	Blunted	Unknown	Unknown	Normal	Blunted	Normal

Appendix 6

Neuroimaging findings in psychiatric disorders

Test	Depression	Bipolar affective disorder, manic	Schizophrenia	Eating disorder	Chronic alcohol dependency	OCD	Alzheimer's disease
Microscopic and molecular anomalies	Unknown	Unknown	Reduced Temporal lobe synaptophysin	Unknown	Punctate lesions of mamillary bodies	Unknown	Senile plaque NFTs Granulovacuolar lesion Hirano bodies
Basal ganglia structure	Atrophy (inconsistent)	Atrophy	Inconsistent	Normal	Normal (except fetal alcohol syndrome)	Atrophy	Atrophy
Basal ganglia function	Increased metabolism	Inconsistent	Normal	Normal	Normal (except severe delirium tremens)	**Increased metabolism**	Hypometabolism
Ventricular structure	Enlarged (mild)	Enlarged (mild)	**Enlarged (moderate)**	Enlarged (reversible)	Enlarged (reversible)	Normal	Enlarged (severe)
Cortical structure	Atrophy (mild)	Atrophy (mild)	Atrophy (moderate)	Atrophy (reversible)	**Atrophy (severe)**	Normal	Atrophy (severe)
Hippocampal stucture	Atrophy (mild)	Unknown	Pyramidal cell disarray	Unknown	Atrophy	Unknown	**Atrophy (severe)**
Frontal lobe function	Hypometabolism	Hypometabolism	Hypometabolism	Unknown	Hypometabolism	Normal	Hypometabolism
White matter lesions	**Increased**	Increased	Normal	Normal	Normal	Normal	Increased

Core feature **emboldened** (where known)

Appendix 7

Cell membrane second messengers

	Hormones	Neurotransmitters	AA
Increases cAMP	ACTH, TSH, LH/FSH PTH, Calcitonin Glucagon G_2, Vasopressin V_2	Adrenergic β_1, β_2 $5HT_4$, $5HT_6$, $5HT_7$ Dopamine D_1, D_5 Histamine H_2	
Decreases cAMP	Opioids Somatostatin	Adrenergic α_2 $5HT_{1abd}$ Acetylcholine muscarinic receptor M_1, M_2 Dopamine D_2, D_3, D_4	
Calcium	LHRH, TRH Vasopressin V_1, Angiotensin	Histamine H_1	
Inositol kinase	Insulin Growth factors		
Ion Channel		Acetylcholine nicotinic receptor $5HT_3$	GABA Glycine Glutamate

Appendix 8

Compendium of neuropsychological tests

Function	Test	Regional basis
Summary measures	Premorbid IQ (NART) Wechsler verbal IQ Wechsler non-verbal performance IQ Mini-mental state examination	Global

Attention and working memory
  Articulatory Loop
 	
  Visuospatial sketch pad
  Central executive
	
	Phonological similarity effect
	Word length effect
	Forward digit span
	Forward block sequence span
	Backward digit span
	Backward block sequence span
	Letter cancellation test
		Multimodal association areas

Response times and psychomotor speed	Tower of London (subscale)	Basal ganglia
Executive functions Planning	 Tower of London Verbal fluency Motor sequencing Trail making test Wisconsin card sorting test	Frontal lobe
Language	Boston naming test	Parietal lobe (dominant)
Visuospatial	Rey–Osterrieth figure	Parietal lobe (non-dominant)

Memory – Explicit
  Immediate free recall
  Delayed recall
  Verbal
  Visual
	
	Paired word recall
	Prose passage recall
	Wechsler, logical memory
	Wechsler, visual memory
		Temporal Lobe (medial)

Memory – Implicit Recognition memory	 Paired word recognition	Basal ganglia

Further reading

Standard textbooks

It is important to select a suitable standard text that covers most of the subject matter in one volume. These books will have to be read repeatedly and essentially learnt, particularly for their clinical content. You only need **one book** and this should be one with which you are comfortable, that is, one which you find easy to read and understand.

Companion to Psychiatric Studies: Kendell and Zealley. Sixth edition. 1998. Churchill Livingstone.
The Essentials of Postgraduate Psychiatry: Murray, Hill and McGuffin. Third edition. 1997. Cambridge University Press.
Oxford Textbook of Psychiatry: Gelder, Gath, Mayou and Cowen. Third edition. 1996. Oxford University Press.

All three of these texts are excellent in terms of style and content, however, our choice would be *Companion to Psychiatric Studies*.

Psychopathology texts

Choose **one** only. Although the oldest one of these books is arguably the best, the most recent is most easily available and possibly the most relevant to current examinations and practice.

Symptoms in the Mind: Sims. Second edition. 1995. Saunders.
Psychopathology: Its causes and symptoms: revised edition. Kraupl-Taylor. 1979. Quatermaine House.
Fish's Clinical Psychopathology. Signs and Symptoms in Psychiatry: Revised reprint. Hamilton. 1974. Wright.

Basic sciences texts

Each of these books has different strengths. Examine all of them but be selective. Choose **one**.

Biological Psychiatry: Trimble. 1996. Wiley. (Most up to date).
Seminars in Basic Neurosciences: Morgan and Butler. 1993. Gaskell. (Easiest to use.)
Scientific Basis of Psychiatry: Weller and Eysenck. 1992. Saunders. (Classic text.)

Additional texts

These can be used for reference purposes but will be needed relatively frequently.

An Introduction to Medical Statistics: Bland. 1995. Oxford Medical Publications.

Drug Treatment in Psychiatry: Silverstone and Turner. Fifth edition. 1995. Routledge.

British National Formulary: Latest edition. (An essential text.)

Introduction to Psychology: Atkinson, Atkinson, Smith and Bem. Eleventh edition. 1993. Harcourt Brace.

Introduction to Psychotherapy: Brown and Peddar. Second edition. 1991. Routledge.

Reference texts

These are useful texts but probably not worth investing in for the purposes of the examination and should be used for clarification and further reading.

Organic Psychiatry: Lishman. Third edition. 1998. Blackwell Science.

An Introduction to Neuroendocrinology: Brown. 1994. Cambridge.

Schizophrenia and Related Syndromes: McKenna. 1994. Oxford.

Handbook of Affective Disorders: Paykel. Second edition. 1992. Churchill Livingstone.

The Management of Depression: Checkley. 1997. Blackwell Science.

Neuropsychology, A Clinical Approach: Walsh. 1994. Churchill Livingstone.

Comprehensive Textbook of Psychiatry: Kaplan and Sadock. Sixth edition. 1995. Williams and Wilkins.

Index

The Multiple Choice Question in Psychiatry Series

- *This series* is designed to prepare candidates for all three multiple choice question papers in the MRCPsych examination. Each book covers one paper and, in presenting a wide range of practice questions, they aim to teach as much as to test.

- *Questions* are arranged as mock examination papers. They are relevant to the syllabus and are based on accessible sources, including standard textbooks and key papers, many from the recommended reading list of the Royal College of Psychiatrists. Explanations, notes and references support most answers. ICD-10 and DSM-IV have been adopted.

- *Highly practical guidance* is offered on preparing for and sitting the exams. This includes detailed advice on organizing revision and developing the expertise and skills to answer MCQs. In addition, the nature of the exams, the regulations and the principles underlying the construction of MCQs are clearly explained.

MCQs for the MRCPsych Part I: Examination
Jane Marshall
0 7506 1871 X   230pp   216 x 138mm   Paperback   Autumn 1995   £18.99

MCQs for the MRCPsych Part II: Clinical Topics Examination
Roger Howells
0 7506 1869 8   314pp   216 x 138mm   Paperback   Autumn 1995   £18.99

FORTHCOMING
MCQs for the MRCPsych Part II: Basic Sciences
Gin Malhi
07506 4089 8   208pp   216 x 138mm   Paperback   Autumn 1999   £17.99

Butterworth-Heinemann books are available from your local bookseller or direct from either our Customer Services Department, Tel: 01865 888180, Fax: 01865 314290 or our website at: http://www.bh.com

Examination Notes in Psychiatry:
A Postgraduate Text
Third edition

Peter Buckley MB Bch BAO
Associate Professor of psychiatry, University Hospital of Cleveland, USA.

Jonathan Bird BSc MB ChB MRCPsych
Consultant Neuro-Psychiatrist, Burden Neurological Hospital, Stapleton, Bristol, UK

Glynn Harrison MB ChB MRCPsych
Consultant Psychiatrist, Nottingham Healthcare Unit, University Hospital, Queen's Medical Centre, Nottingham, UK.

Examination Notes in Psychiatry continues to be a popular postgraduate text and aide-mémoire. It is aimed at psychiatrists in training but will also prove invaluable to all psychiatrists and related mental health professionals who are seeking an up-to-date and comprehensive resource for personal revision and lecture preparation.

- Very substantial revision incorporating recent advances
- Extensive literature review citing up-to-date key references
- ICD-10 and DSM-IV
- Remains a key revision aid and a comprehensive review of psychiatry

Review from *British Journal of Psychiatry*
'... *contains a mine of information in the form of definitions, key facts, figures and lists ... fulfils the need for clarity and accuracy admirably ... those of us who have already passed the examination will regularly return to it for teaching preparation and reference.*'

0 7506 1427 7   216 x 138 mm   Paperback   Autumn 1995   £22.50

Butterworth-Heinemann books are available from your local bookseller or direct from either our Customer Services Department, Tel: 01865 888180, Fax: 01865 314290 or our website at: http://www.bh.com

Postgraduate Psychiatry:
Clinical and Scientific Foundations

Louis Appleby BSc, MRCP, MRCPsych
Senior Lecturer, Department of Psychiatry, University of Manchester,
Withington Hospital, Manchester, UK

David Forshaw MRCPsych, DHMSA, DPMSA
Researcher, Department of Forensic Psychiatry, Institute of Psychiatry,
University of London and Senior Registrar, Maudsley Hospital, London

The ideal companion for all membership candidates for the
MRCPsych and students on masters degrees in psychiatry. It
is designed to be used throughout the training years as a
one-stop course text, full of information that closely follows
the syllabus for the exam.

- Impressively wide-ranging content, yet concisely written to
  aid focused study
- Edited by well respected and experienced clinicians
- Includes a section on the exam itself - how to prepare and
  techniques

0 7506 0488 4   530pp   234 x 156mm   Paperback   Summer
1990   £50.00